Hepatic Encephalopathy

Editor

SAMMY SAAB

CLINICS IN
LIVER DISEASE

www.liver.theclinics.com

Consulting Editor
NORMAN GITLIN

May 2024 • Volume 28 • Number 2

ELSEVIER

1600 John F. Kennedy Boulevard • Suite 1800 • Philadelphia, Pennsylvania, 19103-2899

http://www.theclinics.com

CLINICS IN LIVER DISEASE Volume 28, Number 2
May 2024 ISSN 1089-3261, ISBN-13: 978-0-443-12141-8

Editor: Kerry Holland
Developmental Editor: Akshay Samson

Clinics in Liver Disease (ISSN 1089-3261) is published quarterly by Elsevier Inc., 360 Park Avenue South, New York, NY 10010-1710. Months of issue are February, May, August, and November. Business and Editorial Offices: 1600 John F. Kennedy Blvd., Ste. 1800, Philadelphia, PA 19103-2899. Customer Service Office: 3251 Riverport Lane, Maryland Heights, MO 63043. Periodicals postage paid at New York, NY and additional mailing offices. Subscription prices are $339.00 per year (U.S. individuals), $100.00 per year (U.S. student/resident), $447.00 per year (international individuals), $200.00 per year (international student/resident), $405.00 per year (Canadian individuals), $100.00 per year (Canadian student/resident). For institutional access pricing please contact Customer Service via the contact information below. Foreign air speed delivery is included in all *Clinics* subscription prices. All prices are subject to change without notice. **POSTMASTER:** Send address changes to *Clinics in Liver Disease*, Elsevier Health Sciences Division, Subscription Customer Service, 3251 Riverport Lane, Maryland Heights, MO 63043. **Customer Service: Telephone: 1-800-654-2452 (U.S. and Canada); 314-447-8871 (outside U.S. and Canada). Fax: 314-447-8029. E-mail: journalscustomerservice-usa@ elsevier.com (for print support); journalsonlinesupport-usa@elsevier.com (for online support).**

Reprints. For copies of 100 or more of articles in this publication, please contact the Commercial Reprints Department, Elsevier Inc., 360 Park Avenue South, New York, NY 10010-1710. Tel.: 212-633-3874; Fax: 212-633-3820; E-mail: reprints@elsevier.com.

Clinics in Liver Disease is covered in *MEDLINE/PubMed (Index Medicus)*, Science Citation Index Expanded, Journal Citation Reports/Science Edition, and Current Contents/Clinical Medicine.

Contributors

CONSULTING EDITOR

NORMAN GITLIN, MD, FRCP (London), FRCPE (Edinburgh), FAASLD, FACP, FACG
Head of Hepatology, Southern California Liver Centers, San Clemente, California

EDITOR

SAMMY SAAB, MD, MPH
Departments of Medicine and Surgery, David Geffen School of Medicine at UCLA, Los Angeles, California

AUTHORS

DAVID BERNSTEIN, MD
Professor of Medicine, NYU Grossman School of Medicine, Director, GI and Liver Ambulatory Network-Long Island, NYU Langone Health, New York, New York

ROBERT S. BROWN Jr, MD, MPH
Vincent Astor Distinguished Professor of Medicine and Division Chief, Division of Gastroenterology and Hepatology, NewYork-Presbyterian, Weill Cornell Medical College, New York, New York

ADAM P. BUCKHOLZ, MD, MS
Assistant Professor, Division of Gastroenterology and Hepatology, NewYork-Presbyterian, Weill Cornell Medical College, New York, New York

ALEXANDER CHEN, MD
Resident Physician, Internal Medicine, Robert Wood Johnson Medical School, Rutgers Biomedical and Health Sciences (RBHS), Rutgers University, New Brunswick, New Jersey

GINA CHOI, MD
Associate Professor, Department of Medicine, Professor, Department of Surgery, University of California at Los Angeles, Los Angeles, California

R. TODD FREDERICK, MD
Hepatologist, Division of Hepatology, Department of Advanced Organ Therapies, California Pacific Medical Center, San Francisco, California

DEVIKA GANDHI, MD
Physician, Department of Gastroenterology, Loma Linda University, Loma Linda, California

HUMBERTO C. GONZALEZ, MD
Associate Professor, Division of Gastroenterology and Hepatology, Henry Ford Health, Wayne State University, School of Medicine, Detroit, Michigan

STUART C. GORDON, MD
Professor, Division of Gastroenterology and Hepatology, Henry Ford Health, Wayne State University, School of Medicine, Detroit, Michigan

STEVEN-HUY HAN, MD
Professor, Departments of Medicine and Surgery, University of California at Los Angeles, Los Angeles, California

KEVIN B. HARRIS, MD
Fellow, Division of Gastroenterology and Hepatology, Henry Ford Health, Detroit, Michigan

BRITTNEY IBRAHIM, BS
Researcher, Department of Surgery, University of California at Los Angeles, Los Angeles, California

ALI KHALESSI, MD
Fellow, Rutgers New Jersey School of Medicine, Newark, New Jersey

NYAN LATT, MD
Transplant Hepatologist, Virtua Health System, Center for Liver Disease and Transplant Program, Cherry Hill, New Jersey

EDWARD WOLFGANG LEE, MD, PhD
Professor, Division of Interventional Radiology, Department of Radiology, Division of Liver and Pancreas Transplant Surgery, Department of Surgery, UCLA Medical Center, David Geffen School of Medicine at UCLA, Los Angeles, California

FRANCES LEE, MD
Fellow, Department of Gastroenterology, California Pacific Medical Center, San Francisco, California

SUSAN LEE, PharmD, MBA
Senior Director, Northwell Health Office of Access Strategy, Melville, New York

JUSTINE J. LIANG, MD, MS
Physician, Department of Anesthesiology, UCLA Medical Center, David Geffen School of Medicine at UCLA, Los Angeles, California

EMILY LIN, MD
Physician, Department of Gastroenterology, Loma Linda University, Loma Linda, California

SALIMA S. MAKHANI, MD, MSc
Resident, Zucker School of Medicine at Hofstra/Northwell, Manhasset, New York

GRIFFIN P. McNAMARA, MD
Resident Physician, Division of Interventional Radiology, Department of Radiology, UCLA Medical Center, David Geffen School of Medicine at UCLA, Los Angeles, California

CARLOS MINACAPELLI, MD
Hepatology Researcher, Division of Gastroenterology and Hepatology, Rutgers Robert Wood Johnson Medical School, Center for Liver Diseases and Masses, New Brunswick, New Jersey

SANTIAGO J. MUNOZ, MD, FACP, FACG, FAASLD
Associate Professor, Division of Gastroenterology and Hepatology, Department of Medicine, Johns Hopkins School of Medicine and Medical Institutions, Baltimore, Maryland

KABIRU OHIKERE, MD, MHA
Value-Based Care Coordinator, Value Based Care Department, San Francisco Health Network, Zuckerberg San Francisco General Hospital and Trauma Center, San Francisco, California

NIKOLAOS T. PYRSOPOULOS, MD, PhD, MBA, FACP, AGAF, FAASLD, FRCP
Professor and Chief, Rutgers New Jersey School of Medicine, Newark, New Jersey

RACHEL REDFIELD, MD
Fellow in Transplant Hepatology, Division of Gastroenterology, Resident, Cooper University Hospital, Philadelphia, Pennsylvania

VINOD RUSTGI MD, MBA
Professor, Division of Gastroenterology and Hepatology, Rutgers Robert Wood Johnson Medical School, Center for Liver Diseases and Masses, New Brunswick, New Jersey

ELENA G. SAAB
Medical Doctor Candidate, School of Medicine, Wake Forest University, Winston Salem, North California

AKSHAY SHETTY, MD
Assistant Professor, Department of Medicine, Physician, Department of Surgery, University of California at Los Angeles, Los Angeles, California

JASLEEN SINGH, MD
Clinical Instructor, Department of Medicine, University of California at Los Angeles, Los Angeles, California

CHRISTOPHER TAIT, MD
Gastroenterologist, Division of Gastroenterology and Hepatology, Rutgers Robert Wood Johnson Medical School, New Brunswick, New Jersey

MICHAEL VOLK, MD, MSc
Chair, Department of Medicine, Baylor Scott and White, Central Texas Region, Temple, Texas

ROBERT J. WONG, MD, MS
Clinical Associate Professor, Division of Gastroenterology and Hepatology, Stanford University School of Medicine, Stanford; Gastroenterology Section, Veterans Affairs Palo Alto Healthcare System, Palo Alto, California

Contents

> Hepatic encephalopathy (HE) is a neuropsychiatric syndrome that is observed primarily in patients with liver disease. The pathophysiology is complex and involves many factors including ammonia toxicity, dysregulation of central nervous system activity, and excess inflammatory cytokines. Symptoms of HE range from subclinical to debilitating. HE can be difficult to treat and represents a large burden to patients, their caregivers, and the health-care system because of associated resource utilization. This review article provides an overview of the current understanding of the pathophysiology behind HE and where the current research and treatments are pointing toward.

> Hepatic encephalopathy (HE) remains both a clinical diagnosis and one of exclusion. Laboratory testing is largely focused on identifying precipitating factors. Ammonia levels in the blood can be helpful for the diagnosis of HE but are not required for confirmation. More recent literature is lending support to the prognostic capabilities of ammonia in cirrhosis, both in predicting future HE events and in determining outcomes in hospitalized patients. Accurate ammonia testing requires strict protocols to avoid common pitfalls in the measurement of this labile analyte. Future studies investigating the utility of other laboratory testing to diagnose, stage, or predict HE are encouraged.

> Minimal hepatic encephalopathy (MHE) is a pervasive frequent complication of cirrhosis of any etiology. The diagnosis of MHE is difficult as the standard neurologic examination is essentially within normal limits. None of the symptoms and signs of overt HE is present in a patient with MHE, such as confusion, disorientation, or asterixis. Progress has been made in diagnostic tools for detection of attention and cognitive deficits at the point of care of MHE. The development of MHE significantly impacts quality of life and activities of daily life in affected patients including driving motor vehicles and machine operation.

> Hepatic encephalopathy (HE) can occur as a complication of chronic liver disease as well as acute liver failure. HE is associated with significantly increased morbidity and worse patient outcomes. The clinical manifestation of HE ranges from early less-severe presentations that may only be

accurately detected on dedicated psychomotor diagnostic testing to overt alterations in cognition and mental status to the most severe form of coma. Greater awareness of the clinical manifestations of HE across the spectrum of symptom severity is critical for early identification and timely initiation of appropriate therapy to improve patient outcomes.

treatments discussed provide alternative options for patients who have failed standard of care. However, more high-quality studies are needed to routinely recommend many of these agents.

Hepatic encephalopathy (HE) is a clinically severe and devastating complication of decompensated liver disease affecting mortality, quality of life for patients and families, hospital admission rates, and overall health-care costs globally. Depending on the cause of HE, several medical treatment options have been developed and become available. In some refractory HE, such as spontaneous portosystemic shunt-related HE (SPSS-HE) or posttransjugular intrahepatic portosystemic shunt HE (post-TIPS HE), advanced interventional radiology (IR) procedures have been used, and shown to be effective in these conditions. This review presents 2 effective IR procedures for managing SPSS-HE and post-TIPS HE.

Hepatic encephalopathy, either covert or overt, affects more than half of patients with cirrhosis and has lasting effects even after portal hypertension is corrected. Unfortunately, the current therapeutic options still result in high rates of relapse and progression, in part owing to cost barriers and side effects, leading to poor adherence. This review summarizes emerging treatment options, which could take advantage of alternative disease pathways to improve future care of those with hepatic encephalopathy.

Hepatic encephalopathy is a strong predictor of hospital readmissions in patients with advanced liver disease. The frequent recurrence of hepatic encephalopathy and subsequent readmissions may lead to nonreversible organ dysfunction, resulting in a significant decrease of patient quality of life and increase of health care burden costs for patients and facilities. Many of these readmissions for hepatic encephalopathy are preventable. Multidisciplinary patient-centered care throughout the continuum is essential in the management of hepatic encephalopathy. Understanding the patient's daily functions and limitations in the outpatient setting is key to correctly identifying the cause of hospital admission.

Hepatic encephalopathy (HE) is a strong predictor of early hospital readmission in patients with cirrhosis. Early hospital readmission increases health care costs and is associated with worse survival. Herein we provide an overview of strategies to prevent hospital readmissions in patients with HE, divided into 3 contexts: (a) acute inpatient, (b) immediate postdischarge, and (c) longitudinal outpatient setting.

CLINICS IN LIVER DISEASE

SERIES OF RELATED INTEREST

Gastroenterology Clinics of North America
https://www.gastro.theclinics.com

THE CLINICS ARE AVAILABLE ONLINE!
Access your subscription at:
www.theclinics.com

Preface

Hepatic Encephalopathy

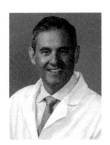

Sammy Saab, MD, MPH
Editor

Hepatic encephalopathy (HE) is an extremely debilitating complication of liver cirrhosis. The basis for the development of HE stems from the interaction of dysbiosis, sarcopenia, liver insufficiency, and portal hypertension.[1] Precipitants of HE include electrolyte disturbances, renal insufficiency, constipation, infection, gastrointestinal bleeding, and use of select medications. Hepatic encephalopathy is rather unique among other manifestations of liver failure in that it affects not only patients but also their caregivers; leaves a cognitive footprint that can persist even after liver transplantation; is a hallmark that marks the beginning of increased health care utilization; and, in severe cases, can be associated with decreased survival.[2]

Caring for patients with cirrhosis and HE poses a number of challenges. First there are no objective criteria for its diagnosis.[3] The diagnosis of HE is made on clinical grounds. The commonly utilized blood test ammonia is neither specific nor sensitive. There is also a spectrum of clinical manifestations of HE. On the one end of the spectrum is early or covert HE, which can include symptoms as innocuous as reversal of sleep-wake cycle, delaye reaction time, or difficulty with arithmetic. Making a diagnosis of early HE requires a great deal of suspicion and the utility of instruments for detection for subclinical HE that are cumbersome and impractical. On the other end of the spectrm can be confusion and even coma. Lactulose, which is the cornerstone in the treatment of HE, is poorly tolerable, and nonadherence is common.[4] Unfortunately we have not had a new medication approved by the Food and Drug Administration for the treatment of HE since rifaximin was approved over a decade ago. Additional treatments are needed, particularly those with refractory HE.

In this issue of *Clinics in Liver Disease*, we look at the entire gamut of HE. We start with a review of the pathophysiology of HE, and provide a guide toward making a diagnosis. We also review the clinical implications of the earlierst form of HE, covett HE. We discuss how HE overt impacts patient prognosis and a patient's social structure. Equally important, we discuss current, future, nontraditional, and radiologic treatments

Clin Liver Dis 28 (2024) xi–xii
https://doi.org/10.1016/j.cld.2024.02.001
1089-3261/24/Published by Elsevier Inc.

liver.theclinics.com

of HE. Moreover, we examine a number of clnically useful approaches to prevent readmissions.

The treatment of HE can be very rewarding. Quality of life and patient-related outcomes improve; caregiver burden decreases, and there may be a decrease in health care utilization. Patients can once again be members of their community.

DISCLOSURES

Dr S. Saab serves on speakers bureaus for AbbVie, Eisai, Gilead, Intercept, Mallinckrodt, Salix, Takeda; and serves as a consultant for Eisai, Gilead, Mallinckrodt.

Sammy Saab, MD, MPH
David Geffen School of Medicine at UCLA
Departments of Medicine and Surgery
Suite 700
100 Medical Plaza
Los Angeles, CA 90095, USA

E-mail address:
ssaab@mednet.ucla.edu

REFERENCES

1. Vilstrup H, Amodio P, Bajaj J, et al. Hepatic encephalopathy in chronic liver disease: 2014 Practice Guideline by the American Association for the Study of Liver Diseases and the European Association for the Study of the Liver. Hepatology 2014;60:715–35.
2. Yanny B, Winters A, Boutros S, et al. Hepatic encephalopathy challenges, burden, and diagnostic and therapeutic approach. Clin Liver Dis 2019;23:607–23.
3. Frenette CT, Levy C, Saab S. Hepatic encephalopathy-related hospitalizations in cirrhosis: transition of care and closing the revolving door. Dig Dis Sci 2022;67: 1994–2004.
4. Chow KW, Ibrahim BM, Yum JJ, et al. Barriers to lactulose adherence in patients with cirrhosis and hepatic encephalopathy. Dig Dis Sci 2023;68:2389–97.

Pathophysiology of Hepatic Encephalopathy

A Framework for Clinicians

Alexander Chen, MD[a], Christopher Tait, MD[b],
Carlos Minacapelli, MD[b,c], Vinod Rustgi, MD, MBA[b,c],*

KEYWORDS

- Hepatic encephalopathy • Pathophysiology • Ammonia
- Portosystemic encephalopathy

KEY POINTS

- Hepatic encephalopathy (HE) presents with a wide variety of symptoms and represents a significant source of morbidity and mortality with an estimated 5-year survival of 15% after the first bout of overt HE in patients with cirrhosis.
- Also known as portosystemic encephalopathy, this clinical state most commonly develops in the setting of cirrhosis with clinically significant portal hypertension, although acute causes of liver injury, disruptions in portal circulation, and medical shunt devices are other important causes of HE.
- HE presents with a diverse spectrum of neurologic, psychiatric, and musculoskeletal symptoms, which ranges from subtle changes in the sleep–wake cycle in early stages to progressive disorientation, memory impairment, and eventually coma in its most severe stages.
- Asterixis, or flapping tremor, is the most recognized symptom but mood changes such as apathy or irritability can be a part of the clinical syndrome.
- Such cognitive and psychiatric symptoms provide a varying degree of impairment and place patients at risk to a wide range of morbid outcomes including significant reductions in health-related quality of life as well as significantly increased yearly mortality risk.

[a] Internal Medicine, Robert Wood Johnson Medical School, Rutgers Biomedical and Health Sciences (RBHS), Rutgers University, New Brunswick, NJ, USA; [b] Division of Gastroenterology and Hepatology, Rutgers Robert Wood Johnson Medical School, New Brunswick, NJ, USA; [c] Center for Liver Diseases and Masses, Rutgers Robert Wood Johnson Medical School, New Brunswick, NJ, USA
* Corresponding author. Rutgers Robert Wood Johnson School of Medicine One Robert Wood Johnson Place Medical Education Building, New Brunswick, NJ 08901.
E-mail address: vinod.rustgi@rutgers.edu

Clin Liver Dis 28 (2024) 209–224
https://doi.org/10.1016/j.cld.2024.01.002
1089-3261/24/© 2024 Elsevier Inc. All rights reserved.

INTRODUCTION AND CLINICAL BACKGROUND

Hepatic encephalopathy (HE) is a neuropsychiatric condition that can develop in patients with acute and chronic liver disease. It presents with a wide variety of symptoms and represents a significant source of morbidity and mortality with an estimated 5-year survival of 15% after the first bout of overt HE in patients with cirrhosis.[1] Also termed portosystemic encephalopathy, this clinical state most commonly develops in the setting of cirrhosis with clinically significant portal hypertension, although acute causes of liver injury, disruptions in portal circulation, and medical shunt devices are other important causes of HE.[1]

HE presents with a diverse spectrum of neurologic, psychiatric, and musculoskeletal symptoms, which ranges from subtle changes in the sleep–wake cycle in early stages to progressive disorientation, memory impairment, and eventually coma in its most severe stages.[2] Asterixis, or flapping tremor, is the most recognized symptom but mood changes such as apathy or irritability can be a part of the clinical syndrome. These cognitive and psychiatric symptoms provide a varying degree of impairment and place patients at risk for a wide range of morbid outcomes including significant reductions in health-related quality of life as well as significantly increased yearly mortality risk.[3]

HE resists simple classification and diagnosis because it encompasses a wide variety of presenting symptoms with large interobserver discrepancies in evaluating patient behavior. HE is a clinical diagnosis with no standardized serologic testing or imaging modality that easily captures severity. Ammonia is classically associated with HE and can be measured clinically but due to lack of specificity and clear correlation with clinical status, does not on its own allow diagnosis or prognosis of HE in most clinical circumstances.[2] One classification system established by the 11th World Congress of Gastroenterology classifies HE into 4 axes that capture multiple facets of this complex clinical process.[4] These 4 axes include classification by (1) underlying disease process, (2) severity, (3) time course, and (4) precipitating features. Classification by underlying disease and time course is especially crucial because this affects clinical management and highlights important pathophysiologic differences seen in acute versus chronic causes of liver failure. The first feature of HE is based on what underlying disease is present, with type A HE developing in the setting of acute liver failure, type B in the setting of portal-systemic bypass with no intrinsic hepatocellular disease, and type C, which is the most common, in the setting of cirrhosis with portal hypertension or systemic shunting. Several classification schemes for disease severity have been identified, all of which attempt to identify covert or subclinical symptoms as well as more severe encephalopathy ranging to gross impairment and comatose states. The West Haven Criteria (WHC) is commonly used in clinical practice, ranging from 0 (minimal) to 4 (comatose) **Fig. 1**. The subjective nature of these scales has led to the development of several systems to capture severity. How the WHC, International Society of Hepatic Encephalopathy and Nitrogen Metabolism (ISHEN), Hepatic Encephalopathy Scoring Algorithm (HESA), and Clinical Hepatic Encephalopathy Staging Scale (CHESS) grades compare is summarized in **Fig. 1**. The third feature of HE is time course, which is subdivided into episodic, recurrent, or persistent. HE is said to be recurrent when bouts of HE recur within intervals of less than 6 months and is said to be persistent when some manifestation of HE is always present; otherwise, it is said to be episodic. The fourth feature of HE is the presence of any identifiable precipitating factors, which are most commonly infections, overdiuresis, dehydration, electrolyte disorders, and constipation.

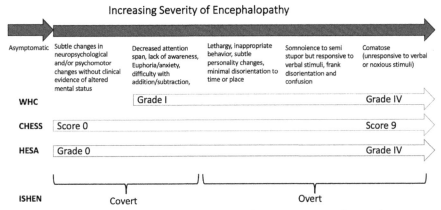

Fig. 1. Assessment Tools for Hepatic Encephalopathy Severity. *Data from* Kabara S, R.V., Hepatic Encephalopathy: A Review. European Medical Journal, 2021. 9: p. 89-97.

Considering the prevalence of HE in advanced liver disease, its broad spectrum of presentation, and highly associated morbidity and mortality, understanding its pathophysiologic underpinning is crucial for clinicians in understanding and managing this condition. Multiple underlying factors including alterations in ammonia homeostasis, altered neurotransmitters, altered nutrient profile, systemic and cerebral inflammation, gut microbiome, and precipitating causes have been implicated in the pathogenesis of HE.[5] This review will describe these pathophysiologic mechanisms and provide a framework for clinicians in the current understanding of this complex condition, as well as emphasis on how these pathologic mechanisms underlie our current clinical treatments.

AMMONIA HOMEOSTASIS AND CHANGES IN LIVER DISEASE
Production, Absorption, and Accumulation

Accumulation of toxic levels of ammonia in the central nervous system (CNS) and systemically has historically been one of the most heavily implicated factors in the pathogenesis of HE.[6] Many other factors are important in the pathogenesis of HE but significant research has shown ammonia plays a central role. The normal physiologic cycle of ammonia involves production and accumulation through breakdown of ingested proteins and subsequent handling by the liver, muscle, and kidneys (**Fig. 2**). The normal physiologic goal of this complex system is to meet the body's demand for nitrogen, which is crucial for amino acid synthesis and energy production, without exposing systemic circulation to toxic levels of ammonia and urea. Because ammonia is a byproduct of the amine group from amino acids, dietary protein is a large source of ammonia. These amine groups are catabolized by bacteria in the gut that have urease and through the action of glutaminase in enterocytes. A large proportion of the body's ammonia is thus formed in the gut by the action of gut bacteria on amino acids, whereas the remainder of systemic ammonia is formed as a byproduct of amino acid handling by the liver, kidney, and skeletal muscle, described in detail in a later section (see **Fig. 2**).

The kidneys play an important role in ammoniagenesis as the site of catabolism of glutamine into bicarbonate and ammonia. The resulting ammonia is either excreted into the urine as the protonated ammonium or returned to systemic circulation, where it is ultimately metabolized by the liver through the urea cycle. Approximately half of

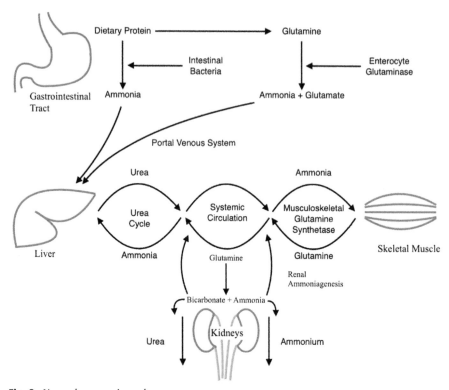

Fig. 2. Normal ammonia cycle.

ammonia generated by the kidneys is excreted in the urine while the other half is returned to systemic circulation.[7] Handling of ammonia by the renal tubules by these mechanisms helps account for the pathophysiology of several HE precipitants, including acidosis, hypokalemia, and hypovolemia. Acidemia promotes renal ammoniagenesis through increased ammonia production to aid in net acid excretion as protonated ammonium. Hypokalemia induces renal ammoniagenesis, although the underlying mechanism is not well understood.[8] Hypokalemia has been found to promote ammonium excretion even when there is a concomitant metabolic alkalosis, worsening the overall acid–base balance.[8] Correcting hypokalemia (if present) is thus an important part of initial HE management. In addition to acid–base and potassium homeostasis, volume status also affects renal ammoniagenesis. Angiotensin II has been shown to upregulate renal ammoniagenesis, which helps explains why low volume states may precipitate HE.[9] Other regulators of renal ammoniagenesis may include prostaglandins, growth hormone, corticosteroids, aldosterone, tricarboxylic acid cycle intermediates and overall tubular flow rate.[10]

Circulation

Ammonia that is produced from the gastrointestinal tract, whether through metabolism by bacteria or enterocytes, then enters the portal venous system and subsequently the liver. The concentration of ammonia in the portal vein can be upward of 10-fold the systemic circulation.[11] Ammonia is metabolized in the liver into urea and transported to the kidneys for excretion (urea cycle, see **Fig. 2**). If the liver is bypassed by a shunt, such as a transjugular intrahepatic portosystemic shunt (TIPS) or a vascular shunt, type

B HE can occur as the high concentrations of ammonia in the portal venous system bypass the liver and cannot be detoxified. Portal hypertension with significant collateral circulation also causes ammonia accumulation as seen in cirrhosis. Ammonia entering the systemic circulation can also be taken up by skeletal muscle that have glutamine synthetase and then be converted into glutamine. Approximately one-third of all nitrogen derived from protein catabolism is transported systemically as glutamine.[12]

Detoxification and Excretion

The majority of ammonia is metabolized into water-soluble urea through the urea cycle (Krebs-Henseleit cycle), which consists of 5 enzymes found in the liver. Inherited disorders of the urea cycle, most commonly ornithine transcarbamylase deficiency, are rare and contribute to a minority of HE cases. Skeletal muscle is an important site of ammonia detoxification. There is increasing evidence that branched chain amino acids (BCAAs) play an important role in augmenting skeletal muscle detoxification of ammonia. It has been shown that in patients with cirrhosis and reduced plasma concentrations of BCAAs with concomitant elevated levels of aromatic amino acids have more severe HE.[13] A recent Cochrane meta-analysis showed BCAA supplementation can help reduce severity of HE symptoms but did not have an effect on mortality.[14] It is hypothesized that BCAAs can help treat HE by preventing muscle loss and by preventing aromatic amino acids from crossing the blood–brain barrier.[15]

There has been recent evidence that supplementation with L-ornithine L-aspartate (LOLA), which is a stable salt of the amino acids ornithine and aspartate, both improves symptoms of HE and decreases short-term mortality. These amino acids act as substrates for enzymes in the urea cycle and for glutamine synthetase, increasing their activity and consumption of ammonia.[16] A recent double-blind randomized controlled trial showed that LOLA combined with lactulose and rifaximin led to lower ammonia levels, faster recovery from HE and lower 28 day mortality compared with lactulose and rifaximin plus placebo.[17] This study also showed that the addition of LOLA led to lower levels of systemic interleukin (IL)-6 and tumor necrosis factor alpha (TNF-α), which correlates with evidence that these cytokines likely play a key role in the pathophysiology of HE.

The most commonly used clinical treatments for HE rely on aiding gut excretion of ammonia, most commonly achieved with oral lactulose. Lactulose is a disaccharide that cannot be metabolized by the small intestines. Once reaching the colon, lactulose is catabolized by bacteria into short-chain fatty acids that lower colonic pH. This acidic environment traps ammonia in the colon as protonated ammonium, which is then excreted. Lactulose also promotes the growth of nonurease producing *Lactobacillus* bacteria[18] and its osmotic laxative effect decreases colonic transit time, which leads to less time for ammonia to be absorbed. Lactulose has been shown to have significant improvement in treating symptoms of HE in cirrhosis, although does not improve overall mortality.[19] Lactulose use is controversial in the setting of acute liver failure because trials have not demonstrated a significant improvement in mortality or improvement in encephalopathy and often causes significant abdominal distention, which can complicate liver transplant.[20]

The Role of Skeletal Muscle

Patients with HE have historically been placed on protein-restricted diets in an attempt to limit ammonia accumulation from dietary proteins. Recent clinical evidence, however, suggests that protein-restricted diets can worsen HE, likely because these diets exacerbate sarcopenia and skeletal muscle is an important source of ammonia meta-bolism for patients with liver disease.[12,21,22] Skeletal muscle can uptake ammonia and convert it to glutamine which can be used for protein synthesis and nucleotide synthe-sis. The critical ammonia-detoxifying role of skeletal muscle in patients with HE may also help to explain the therapeutic benefit of BCAA supplementation. It is hypothe-sized that BCAA supplementation can help prevent skeletal muscle loss and promote synthesis of glutamine from ammonia in skeletal muscle.[15]

Liver dysfunction and ammonia accumulation: In liver dysfunction such as cirrhosis, progressive damage to and loss of hepatocytes causes decreased ability to detoxify ammonia into urea or glutamine, and increasing portal hypertension causes progres-sively increasing portosystemic bypass whereby collateral vessels are increasingly relied on for venous return. This leads to the accumulation of ammonia in the systemic circulation to toxic levels that can affect the CNS.[23] Other causes of portal hyperten-sion lead to portosystemic bypass of liver ammonia detoxification, which includes presinusoidal or postsinusoidal causes of portal hypertension including portal vein thrombosis or Budd-Chiari syndrome. Increased ammonia absorption can also occur when there is more ammonia available such as with proliferation of pathogenic urease containing bacteria or increased dietary intake. Furthermore, decreased colonic transit time as occurs in constipation can provide more time for absorption, high-lighting constipation (particularly in the setting of opioid use) as a common precipitant. In patients with acute on chronic liver disease there is usually a trigger which precip-itates HE but ammonia levels vary greatly among patients with HE and have been found to frequently be unreliable. In acute liver failure, arterial ammonia levels corre-late more closely with degree of HE severity and are a poor prognostic factor high-lighting how in cases of acute liver failure there are less compensatory pathways for ammonia handling than typically seen in chronic cases. Arterial ammonia levels are also correlated with degree of cerebral herniation and swelling, which is much more severe in acute liver failure than in chronic liver disease where cerebral edema is often subtle.[24,25] In patients with liver disease for whom intrahepatic portosystemic shunt placement is necessary because of high portal pressures, the resultant hepatic bypass can often lead to chronically elevated ammonia levels and worsened or refrac-tory HE.[26]

Clinical Utility of Serum Ammonia Measurement

Despite the central role that ammonia dysregulation plays in the pathophysiology of HE, measuring ammonia levels in patients with HE is of less clinical utility in most set-tings. External factors such as whether a patient's blood is frozen before being pro-cessed, how quickly the sample is placed on ice, and whether they recently had a protein-rich meal before their sample was drawn causes significant variability between samples.[27,28] Serum ammonia is also affected by each individual patient's renal func-tion and muscle mass, and many other sources of elevated ammonia exist including gastrointestinal bleeding, urinary tract infection, and shock.[28] Although there is a gross correlation between severity of HE and measured serum arterial and venous ammonia levels up to elevations two times the upper limit of normal range, there is considerable overlap of ammonia levels observed for different grades of HE.[29] Despite the limited value of measuring ammonia levels in patients with HE, it continues to be a routine clin-ical practice. There is one important exception where measuring ammonia carries clin-ical utility, and that includes cases of acute liver failure particularly due to viral hepatitis. Elevated arterial ammonia in the first 24 hours of presentation has been observed to be a poor prognostic factor.[30] The incorporation of ammonia levels into prognostication or severity scoring system requires further investigation, and its use in routine clinical practice in patients with chronic liver disease should be more heavily scrutinized.

PATHOLOGIC EFFECTS OF EXCESS AMMONIA
Central Nervous System Access

The vast majority of ammonia crosses the blood–brain barrier via simple passive diffusion in the free base form (NH_3). However, it is estimated that up to 25% can diffuse in the protonated form ($+NH_4$).[5] Once inside the CNS where there are no cells that can perform the urea cycle, and astrocytes preferentially take up ammonia as the only brain cell containing glutamine synthase.[31] Ammonia in excess concentrations then impairs astrocyte regulation of pH and potassium concentrations, which in turn interferes with normal inhibitory neurotransmission pathways.[32]

Direct Neurotoxicity

In addition to these biochemical effects, it has been shown that ammonia induces astrocyte swelling by the osmotic activity of glutamine after conversion from ammonia, which is thought to be a key step in the development of HE.[33] However, mouse models have demonstrated that mice exposed to toxic levels of ammonia showed acute astrocyte dysfunction even before swelling occurred, suggesting morphologic changes and swelling are not the only pathogenic mechanism for astrocyte dysfunction.[32] Astrocyte cells exposed to elevated levels of ammonia developed high levels of extracellular potassium, which overactivated the NKCC1 receptor and consequently interfered with the inhibitory effect of gamma-aminobutyric acid (GABA). This new finding also has important implications for therapy because studies have shown that bumetanide, a specific NKCC1 receptor inhibitor, attenuated cortical dysfunction and improved survival in animal models.[32]

Cerebral Edema

Regardless of where specifically in the causal chain astrocyte swelling plays a role in precipitating HE, generalized cerebral edema has been observed in patients with liver disease and is thought to play a role in HE.[25,34] MRI studies have shown cerebral edema in patients with HE that worsens with increasing HE severity, such as after a TIPS procedure and has been shown to resolve after liver transplantation or medical treatment of HE.[34] Multiple mechanisms have been implicated in the pathophysiology of this edema. As described previously in relation to direct neurotoxicity, osmotically active glutamine accumulates as astrocytes detoxify ammonia. Ammonia also triggers an oxidative stress response in astrocytes with the activation of the N-methyl-D-aspartate (NMDA) glutamate receptors playing a key role. The exact mechanism is unclear; however, it seems NMDA activation is both precipitated by and a causal factor for astrocyte swelling, suggesting a possible self-induced feedback loop.[34] It has been observed that NMDA inhibitors can decrease swelling in rats exposed to ammonia toxicity.[33] Specifically, memantine has been shown to provide some benefit in improving HE symptoms in animal models.[35] Other metabolic derangements can also contribute to cerebral edema, most notably hyponatremia.

NEUROTRANSMITTER DYSFUNCTION
Gamma-aminobutyric Acid

GABA is the main inhibitory neurotransmitter in the CNS. It has long been thought that patients with HE have increased "GABAergic tone" based on animal models with hepatic failure.[36] This lead to the use of the GABA receptor antagonist flumazenil in patients with HE, which has been called into question recently given the lack of high-quality evidence to suggest it improves outcomes.[37] However, it has been demonstrated that both acute and chronic liver failure leads to increased expression of the 18-kDa translocator protein.[38] Activation of the 18-kDA protein has been shown to lead to de novo synthesis of neurosteroids such as allopregnanolone that can contribute to neuroinhibition.[39] Allopregnanolone can readily cross the blood-brain barrier and promotes the binding of GABA and benzodiazepines to their respective receptors, possibly offering a link between increased "GABAergic tone" in patients with HE and increased ammonia.[38] GR3027, a new selective antagonist of neurosteroids, has shown promise in treating symptoms of HE.[40,41]

Glutamate

Glutamate is the main excitatory neurotransmitter of the nervous system. When it accumulates in excess, it is normally taken up by astrocytes and converted to glutamine, which can be returned to neurons and recycled back into glutamate. In patients with elevated ammonia levels, glutamate transporter expression is impaired, which prevents this normal recycling and causes glutamate to accumulate in synaptic clefts leading to overexcitation.[42] This in turn leads to greater NMDA activation and oxidative and nitrosative stress.[38] However, after chronic exposure to elevated ammonia levels, glutamate receptor expression seems to normalize.[42,43]

Monoamines

Important signaling monoamines include the neurotransmitters histamine, serotonin, and dopamine. Elevated levels of histamine have been found in patients with HE and is hypothesized to contribute to sleep pattern disturbances as well as disturbed movement patterns.[43] Increased levels of serotonin metabolites in the cerebrospinal fluid of patients who died of hepatic comas suggest high turnover of serotonin.[44] This leads to a decrease in the amount of overall available serotonin, which can contribute to the neuropsychiatric symptoms of HE.[45] Increased activity of dopamine metabolizing enzymes and downregulation of dopamine receptors leading to overall decreased dopaminergic tone has been noted in animal models, which is thought to contribute to motor and psychiatric disturbances of HE.[46] However, levodopa and bromocriptine have not been shown to improve mortality or outcomes in HE.[47]

CHRONIC INFECTION AND INFLAMMATION
Pathogenic Features of Intestinal Bacteria in Liver Disease

Although acute infection is a common precipitant of HE, there is copious evidence that patients with cirrhosis are in a state of chronic low level infection from gut bacterial translocation, which induces systemic inflammation that can predispose patients to HE.[48] One theorized mechanism is that the vascular congestion and mucosal edema that follows increased portal pressure facilitates increased translocation of pathogenic bacteria. However, this has not been well validated because portal hypertension without liver insufficiency has not been shown to lead to bacterial translocation, whereas animal models with liver insufficiency and normal portal pressure do have increased incidence of translocated bacteria.[49] Another key contributor to bacterial translocation and chronic infection in patients with liver disease is disruption of the gut microbiota. It is hypothesized that changes in intestinal dysmotility, gastric tract pH, and disruption in production of bile acids in advanced liver disease all lead to gut dysbiosis that facilitates translocation of harmful bacteria.[13,50] One theorized mechanism proposes that decreased bile acid production allows overproliferation of urease-producing bacteria such as Lachnospiraceae.[51] In addition to inflammation induced by gut translocation of bacteria, a recent animal model showed rats were fed an ammonia-rich diet developed increased levels of inflammatory cytokines including TNF-α, IL-6, IL-10, and Prostaglandin E2 (PGE2) that was reversible when ammonia levels normalized. They also demonstrated that the reversal of peripheral inflammation with infliximab prevented cognitive decline while the rats still had elevated ammonia levels, suggesting peripheral inflammation is a crucial link between elevated ammonia levels and central effects.[52]

Gut Dysbiosis

There is increasing evidence that gut dysbiosis plays a key role in HE by mediating systemic inflammation. The gut microbiome in patients with cirrhosis and HE demonstrates significant differences to those with no cognitive impairment. An overgrowth of more pathogenic urease positive bacteria such as *Enterococcus* and *Burkholderia* has been correlated with worsened cognition in those with HE while the presence of normal autochthonous flora is associated with improved cognition.[13] A concomitant increase in systemic inflammatory cytokines has been found in those that have gut dysbiosis.[53,54] Because there is strong evidence for dysbiosis as an important factor in HE, there has been increased interest in probiotics as a treatment to restore normal gut homeostasis and reduce systemic inflammation by decreasing bacterial urease activity, bacterial translocation, and ammonia absorption. Recent metanalyses suggest probiotics are superior to placebo in treating HE but are not more efficacious than lactulose.[13] In addition to probiotics, recent evidence has emerged for the use of fecal transplant to treat gut dysbiosis in patients with HE. Bajaj and colleagues performed the first randomized controlled trial to demonstrate the efficacy of fecal transplant in which 20 patients with recurrent HE were randomized to fecal transplant enemas or lactulose. Those in the fecal transplant group had fewer adverse effects, fewer bouts of HE and fewer hospitalizations at 1 year follow-up when compared with the control group.[55] Bajaj and colleagues later showed in a placebo controlled trial that capsular preparations of donor fecal bacteria were safe, well tolerated and reduced dysbiosis; however, the study was too small to detect efficacy.[56]

Given the role of pathogenic glut flora in HE, antibiotic therapy is a mainstay of HE treatment with rifaximin being the most commonly used because of its poor systemic absorption.[16] Rifaximin is a broad-spectrum antibiotic with anerobic coverage, which has been shown to be effective in treating HE without increase in adverse effects such as *Clostridium difficile* infection or increased antibiotic resistance.[57,58] Some medications impact the gut flora negatively and can worsen dysbiosis and increase HE risk. A recent meta-analysis found that the use of proton pump inhibitors (PPIs) was correlated with an increased risk for HE in patients with liver dysfunction.[59] It is still unclear if there is a causal relationship but it is theorized that the change in gut pH caused by PPIs leads to alteration of the gut microbiota and an increased risk for pathogenic bacterial translocation and subsequent infection or increased systemic inflammation. As such, PPIs should be used judiciously in patients with cirrhosis. The many factors and treatments involved in gut homeostasis in HE are summarized in **Fig. 3**.[13]

Tumor Necrosis Factor Alpha Theory

In addition to translocated bacteria and gut dysbiosis, increased levels of TNF-α that have been observed in patients with chronic liver disease may also result from

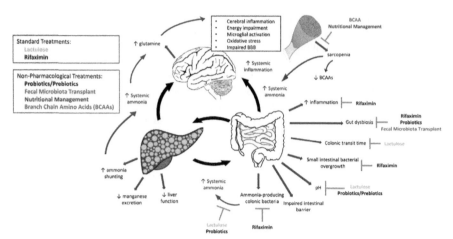

Fig. 3. Treatments for different pathogenic mechanisms of HE. (*Adapted from*: Weir, V. and K.R. Reddy, *Nonpharmacologic Management of Hepatic Encephalopathy: An Update.* Clin Liver Dis, 2020. **24**(2): p. 243-261.)

increased production of TNF-α from Kupffer cells and decreased clearance in individuals with concomitant renal disease.[60] TNF-α levels have been noted to correlate with degree of severity of HE in patients with liver disease, and there are several proposed mechanism to explain this relationship.[61] TNF-α has been shown to facilitate diffusion of ammonia into the CNS allowing for faster accumulation of toxic levels of ammonia.[62] TNF-α has also been linked to brain edema noted in HE, although the exact relationship is unclear. Some explanations include TNF-α's ability to increase microvascular permeability and cause capillary fluid leakage and TNF-α's noted ability to directly cause astrocyte swelling.[60] With respect to neurotransmitter activity, there is also evidence that TNF-α inhibits uptake of glutamate leading to further glutamate toxicity that is noted in HE. The relationship between TNF-α and GABA in HE is not as clear, although evidence shows elevated central GABA levels when TNF-α levels are elevated such as in sepsis[60] (**Fig. 4**).

MICRONUTRIENT AND ELECTROLYTE IMBALANCE

As discussed with regards to dietary protein and BCAAs, there are many nutritional factors that influence the onset of HE. Manganese is a trace element and essential micronutrient metal that can accumulate in patients with liver dysfunction because it is normally excreted via the biliary tract and can accumulate with portal-systemic shunting.[63] This excess manganese has been shown to deposit in the globus pallidus, which can be demonstrated on T1 MRI and is thought to contribute to the extrapyramidal symptoms that can be seen in HE.[64] Manganese in the astrocyte disrupts oxidative phosphorylation in the mitochondria and exacerbates oxidative stress. Zinc is an essential micronutrient that is commonly deficient in patients with liver disease.[65] It is a cofactor for enzymes found in the urea cycle, glutamine synthetase, and for the antioxidant enzyme superoxide dismutase. There is some evidence that oral zinc can aid in alleviating neurocognitive deficits when used in conjunction with standard therapies.[66] Thiamine deficiency is commonly found in this population, particularly those with alcoholic liver disease and can confound diagnosis of HE when there is concurrent Wernicke's encephalopathy or Korsakoff syndrome.

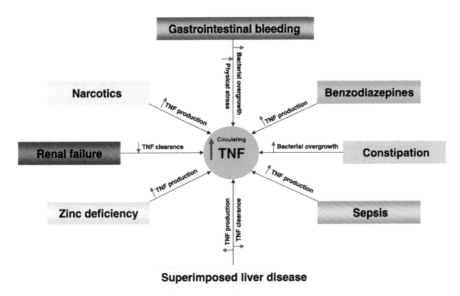

Fig. 4. Factors influencing serum TNF-α levels. (*Adapted from*: Odeh, M., *Pathogenesis of hepatic encephalopathy: the tumour necrosis factor-alpha theory.* Eur J Clin Invest, 2007. **37**(4): p. 291-304.)

Electrolyte imbalances are also a common occurrence in patients with advanced liver disease and hyponatremia in particular plays an important role in the pathophysiology of HE. There are 2 processes by which hyponatremia develops in these patients; hypovolemic patients retain excess solute free water to increase intravascular volume, whereas hypervolemic patients have impaired ability to excrete solute-free water.[67] Recent studies have suggested that hyponatremia in patients with end-stage liver disease is a predictor for the development of overt HE.[68,69] A possible explanation for this relationship is that hyponatremia can induce cerebral edema, which augments or synergistically acts with the ability of ammonia to induce astrocyte swelling.[70] As discussed earlier, regulation of potassium is closely linked to maintaining acid–base homeostasis and allowing proper renal handling of ammonia. Considering how closely related electrolyte and micronutrient regulation is to the development of HE, clinicians should be proactive about addressing imbalances in those are risk of developing HE.

SUMMARY

The pathophysiology of HE is a multiaxis process that involves dysregulation of nitrogen metabolism, the gut microbiota, systemic inflammatory cytokines, CNS structure and function, and micronutrient imbalance. The clinicians approach in thinking about and treating HE should be as encompassing as the underlying process is, considering these various systems, which are all implied in some way. Many of the current treatments for HE have logical mechanistic basis when considering the mechanisms discussed here, and future therapies focus on trialing many of the processes described, including BCAAs, LOLA, and fecal microbiotal transplant. Future research will undoubtedly shed more light on how these processes are connected and are responsible for the development of HE.

CLINICS CARE POINTS

- Lactulose and rifaximin remain the mainstays of treating HE by reducing systemic ammonia
- There is increasing evidence fecal transplant will play a major role in the future for treatment of HE given the pathogenic role of gut dysbiosis
- BCAAs can help reduce symptoms of HE but evidence they improve mortality is more limited
- Checking serum ammonia in patients with HE is of limited clinical utility because of its poor correlation with symptoms and outcomes
- There is a lack of consistent high-quality evidence to support the use of flumazenil in patients with HE despite the role of "increased GABAergic tone" in HE

ACKNOWLEDGMENTS

Author contributions: All authors worked in all 4 aspects of authorship as per ICMJE guidelines.

DISCLOSURE

No conflicts of interest, financial or otherwise, are declared by the authors.
Funding: This study received no external funding.

REFERENCES

1. Elsaid MI, Rustgi VK. Epidemiology of hepatic encephalopathy. Clin Liver Dis 2020;24(2):157–74.
2. Kabara S RV. Hepatic encephalopathy: a review. European Medical Journal 2021; 9:89–97.
3. Dellatore P, Cheung M, Mahpour NY, et al. Clinical Manifestations of Hepatic Encephalopathy. Clin Liver Dis 2020;24(2):189–96.
4. Ferenci P, Lockwood A, Mullen K, et al. Hepatic encephalopathy–definition, nomenclature, diagnosis, and quantification: final report of the working party at the 11th World Congresses of Gastroenterology, Vienna, 1998. Hepatology 2002;35(3):716–21.
5. Jaffe A, Lim JK, Jakab SS. Pathophysiology of hepatic encephalopathy. Clin Liver Dis 2020;24(2):175–88.
6. Aldridge DR, Tranah EJ, Shawcross DL. Pathogenesis of hepatic encephalopathy: role of ammonia and systemic inflammation. J Clin Exp Hepatol 2015; 5(Suppl 1):S7–20.
7. Weiner ID, Mitch WE, Sands JM. Urea and ammonia metabolism and the control of renal nitrogen excretion. Clin J Am Soc Nephrol 2015;10(8):1444–58.
8. Weiner ID, Verlander JW. Renal ammonia metabolism and transport. Compr Physiol 2013;3(1):201–20.
9. Nagami GT. Effect of angiotensin II on ammonia production and secretion by mouse proximal tubules perfused in vitro. J Clin Invest 1992;89(3):925–31.
10. Tannen RL, Sahai A. Biochemical pathways and modulators of renal ammonia-genesis. Miner Electrolyte Metab 1990;16(5):249–58.
11. Cordoba J. and A.T. Blei, Hepatic Encephalopathy, In: M.F.S. Eugene R. Schiff, Willis C. Maddrey, Editor. Schiff's Diseases of the Liver, 2003. Lippincott Williams & Wilkins; Philadelphia, PA, 593-623.

12. He Y, Hakvoort TBM, Köhler SE, et al. Glutamine synthetase in muscle is required for glutamine production during fasting and extrahepatic ammonia detoxification. J Biol Chem 2010;285(13):9516–24.
13. Weir V, Reddy KR. Nonpharmacologic management of hepatic encephalopathy: an Update. Clin Liver Dis 2020;24(2):243–61.
14. Gluud LL, et al. Branched-chain amino acids for people with hepatic encephalopathy. Cochrane Database Syst Rev 2017;5(5):CD001939.
15. Holecek M. Three targets of branched-chain amino acid supplementation in the treatment of liver disease. Nutrition 2010;26(5):482–90.
16. Mahpour NY, Pioppo-Phelan L, Reja M, et al. Pharmacologic Management of Hepatic Encephalopathy. Clin Liver Dis 2020;24(2):231–42.
17. Jain A, Sharma BC, Mahajan B, et al. L-ornithine L-aspartate in acute treatment of severe hepatic encephalopathy: A double-blind randomized controlled trial. Hepatology 2022;75(5):1194–203.
18. Riggio O, Varriale M, Testore GP, et al. Effect of lactitol and lactulose administration on the fecal flora in cirrhotic patients. J Clin Gastroenterol 1990;12(4):433–6.
19. Als-Nielsen B, Gluud LL, Gluud C. Nonabsorbable disaccharides for hepatic encephalopathy. Cochrane Database Syst Rev 2004;(2):CD003044.
20. McDowell Torres D, Stevens RD, Gurakar A. Acute liver failure: a management challenge for the practicing gastroenterologist. Gastroenterol Hepatol 2010;6(7):444–50.
21. Córdoba J, López-Hellín J, Planas M, et al. Normal protein diet for episodic hepatic encephalopathy: results of a randomized study. J Hepatol 2004;41(1):38–43.
22. Lattanzi B, D'Ambrosio D, Merli M. Hepatic encephalopathy and sarcopenia: two Faces of the Same metabolic alteration. J Clin Exp Hepatol 2019;9(1):125–30.
23. Häussinger D, Dhiman RK, Felipo V, et al. Hepatic encephalopathy. Nat Rev Dis Primers 2022;8(1):43.
24. Clemmesen JO, Larsen FS, Kondrup J, et al. Cerebral herniation in patients with acute liver failure is correlated with arterial ammonia concentration. Hepatology 1999;29(3):648–53.
25. Häussinger D, Kircheis G, Fischer R, et al. Hepatic encephalopathy in chronic liver disease: a clinical manifestation of astrocyte swelling and low-grade cerebral edema? J Hepatol 2000;32(6):1035–8.
26. Schindler P, Heinzow H, Trebicka J, Wildgruber M. Shunt-Induced Hepatic Encephalopathy in TIPS: Current Approaches and Clinical Challenges. J Clin Med 2020;9(11):3784.
27. Bajaj JS, Bloom PP, Chung RT, et al. Variability and Lability of Ammonia Levels in Healthy Volunteers and Patients With Cirrhosis: Implications for Trial Design and Clinical Practice. Am J Gastroenterol 2020;115(5):783–5.
28. Haj M, Rockey DC. Ammonia levels do not Guide clinical management of patients with hepatic encephalopathy caused by cirrhosis. Am J Gastroenterol 2020;115(5):723–8.
29. Ong JP, Aggarwal A, Krieger D, et al. Correlation between ammonia levels and the severity of hepatic encephalopathy. Am J Med 2003;114(3):188–93.
30. Bhatia V, Singh R, Acharya SK. Predictive value of arterial ammonia for complications and outcome in acute liver failure. Gut 2006;55(1):98–104.

31. Martinez-Hernandez A, Bell KP, Norenberg MD. Glutamine synthetase: glial localization in brain. Science 1977;195(4284):1356–8.
32. Rangroo Thrane V, Thrane AS, Wang F, et al. Ammonia triggers neuronal disinhibition and seizures by impairing astrocyte potassium buffering. Nat Med 2013 Dec;19(12):1643–8.
33. Oja SS, Saransaari P, Korpi ER. Neurotoxicity of ammonia. Neurochem Res 2017; 42(3):713–20.
34. Haussinger D. Low grade cerebral edema and the pathogenesis of hepatic encephalopathy in cirrhosis. Hepatology 2006;43(6):1187–90.
35. Vogels BA, Maas MA, Daalhuisen J, et al. Memantine, a noncompetitive NMDA receptor antagonist improves hyperammonemia-induced encephalopathy and acute hepatic encephalopathy in rats. Hepatology 1997;25(4):820–7.
36. Ahboucha S, Butterworth RF. Pathophysiology of hepatic encephalopathy: a new look at GABA from the molecular standpoint. Metab Brain Dis 2004;19(3–4): 331–43.
37. Goh ET, Andersen ML, Morgan MY, Gluud LL. Flumazenil versus placebo or no intervention for people with cirrhosis and hepatic encephalopathy. Cochrane Database Syst Rev 2017;7(7):CD002798.
38. Butterworth RF. Altered glial-neuronal crosstalk: cornerstone in the pathogenesis of hepatic encephalopathy. Neurochem Int 2010;57(4):383–8.
39. Mellon SH, Griffin LD. Neurosteroids: biochemistry and clinical significance. Trends Endocrinol Metab 2002;13(1):35–43.
40. Johansson M, Agusti A, Llansola M, et al. GR3027 antagonizes GABAA receptor-potentiating neurosteroids and restores spatial learning and motor coordination in rats with chronic hyperammonemia and hepatic encephalopathy. Am J Physiol Gastrointest Liver Physiol 2015;309(5):G400–9.
41. Johansson M, Månsson M, Lins LE, et al. GR3027 reversal of neurosteroid-induced, GABA-A receptor-mediated inhibition of human brain function: an allopregnanolone challenge study. Psychopharmacology (Berl) 2018;235(5): 1533–43.
42. Butterworth RF. Glutamate transporters in hyperammonemia. Neurochem Int 2002;41(2–3):81–5.
43. Palomero-Gallagher N, Zilles K. Neurotransmitter receptor alterations in hepatic encephalopathy: a review. Arch Biochem Biophys 2013;536(2):109–21.
44. Jellinger K, Riederer P, Kleinberger G, et al. Brain monoamines in human hepatic encephalopathy. Acta Neuropathol 1978;43(1–2):63–8.
45. Dantzer R, O'Connor JC, Lawson MA, Kelley KW. Inflammation-associated depression: from serotonin to kynurenine. Psychoneuroendocrinology 2011; 36(3):426–36.
46. Albrecht J, Jones EA. Hepatic encephalopathy: molecular mechanisms underlying the clinical syndrome. J Neurol Sci 1999;170(2):138–46.
47. Junker AE, Als-Nielsen B, Gluud C, Gluud LL. Dopamine agents for hepatic encephalopathy. Cochrane Database Syst Rev 2014;2014(2):CD003047.
48. Tilg H, Wilmer A, Vogel W, et al. Serum levels of cytokines in chronic liver diseases. Gastroenterology 1992;103(1):264–74.
49. Wiest R, Lawson M, Geuking M. Pathological bacterial translocation in liver cirrhosis. J Hepatol 2014;60(1):197–209.
50. Fukui H. Role of gut dysbiosis in liver diseases: what have We Learned So far? Diseases 2019;7(4).

51. Liu Q, Duan ZP, Ha DK, et al. Synbiotic modulation of gut flora: effect on minimal hepatic encephalopathy in patients with cirrhosis. Hepatology 2004;39(5): 1441–9.
52. Balzano T, Dadsetan S, Forteza J, et al. Chronic hyperammonemia induces peripheral inflammation that leads to cognitive impairment in rats: Reversed by anti-TNF-α treatment. J Hepatol 2020;73(3):582–92.
53. Bajaj JS, Ridlon JM, Hylemon PB, et al. Linkage of gut microbiome with cognition in hepatic encephalopathy. Am J Physiol Gastrointest Liver Physiol 2012;302(1): G168–75.
54. Bajaj JS. The role of microbiota in hepatic encephalopathy. Gut Microb 2014;5(3): 397–403.
55. Bajaj JS, Kassam Z, Fagan A, et al. Fecal microbiota transplant from a rational stool donor improves hepatic encephalopathy: A randomized clinical trial. Hepatology 2017;66(6):1727–38.
56. Bajaj JS, Salzman NH, Acharya C, et al. Fecal Microbial Transplant Capsules Are Safe in Hepatic Encephalopathy: A Phase 1, Randomized, Placebo-Controlled Trial. Hepatology 2019;70(5):1690–703.
57. Bass NM, Mullen KD, Sanyal A, et al. Rifaximin treatment in hepatic encephalopathy. N Engl J Med 2010;362(12):1071–81.
58. Mullen KD, Sanyal AJ, Bass NM, et al. Rifaximin is safe and well tolerated for long-term maintenance of remission from overt hepatic encephalopathy. Clin Gastroenterol Hepatol 2014;12(8). 1390–7.e2.
59. Bian J, Wang A, Lin J, Wu L, et al. Association between proton pump inhibitors and hepatic encephalopathy: A meta-analysis. Medicine (Baltimore) 2017; 96(17):e6723.
60. Odeh M. Pathogenesis of hepatic encephalopathy: the tumour necrosis factor-alpha theory. Eur J Clin Invest 2007;37(4):291–304.
61. Odeh M, Sabo E, Srugo I, Oliven A. Serum levels of tumor necrosis factor-alpha correlate with severity of hepatic encephalopathy due to chronic liver failure. Liver Int 2004;24(2):110–6.
62. Duchini A, Govindarajan S, Santucci M, et al. Effects of tumor necrosis factor-alpha and interleukin-6 on fluid-phase permeability and ammonia diffusion in CNS-derived endothelial cells. J Investig Med 1996;44(8):474–82.
63. Rose C, Butterworth RF, Zayed J, et al. Manganese deposition in basal ganglia structures results from both portal-systemic shunting and liver dysfunction. Gastroenterology 1999;117(3):640–4.
64. Butterworth RF, Spahr L, Fontaine S, Layrargues GP. Manganese toxicity, dopaminergic dysfunction and hepatic encephalopathy. Metab Brain Dis 1995;10(4): 259–67.
65. Marchesini G, Fabbri A, Bianchi G, et al. Zinc supplementation and amino acid-nitrogen metabolism in patients with advanced cirrhosis. Hepatology 1996;23(5): 1084–92.
66. Takuma Y, Nouso K, Makino Y, et al. Clinical trial: oral zinc in hepatic encephalopathy. Aliment Pharmacol Ther 2010;32(9):1080–90.
67. Jiménez JV, Carrillo-Pérez DL, Rosado-Canto R, et al. Electrolyte and Acid-Base Disturbances in End-Stage Liver Disease: A Physiopathological Approach. Dig Dis Sci 2017;62(8):1855–71.
68. Guevara M, Baccaro ME, Torre A, et al. Hyponatremia is a risk factor of hepatic encephalopathy in patients with cirrhosis: a prospective study with time-dependent analysis. Am J Gastroenterol 2009;104(6):1382–9.

69. Riggio O, Angeloni S, Salvatori FM, et al. Incidence, natural history, and risk factors of hepatic encephalopathy after transjugular intrahepatic portosystemic shunt with polytetrafluoroethylene-covered stent grafts. Am J Gastroenterol 2008;103(11): 2738–46.
70. Cordoba J, Garcia-Martinez R, Simon-Talero M. Hyponatremic and hepatic encephalopathies: similarities, differences and coexistence. Metab Brain Dis 2010;25(1):73–80.

Hepatic Encephalopathy—A Guide to Laboratory Testing

Frances Lee, MD[a], R. Todd Frederick, MD[b],*

KEYWORDS

- Hepatic encephalopathy • Ammonia • Hyperammonemia • IL-6

KEY POINTS

- Laboratory testing for hepatic encephalopathy (HE) should be tailored to the clinical scenario.
- Blood testing of ammonia is not diagnostic for HE, but it can be helpful in supporting or excluding a diagnosis of HE when in doubt.
- Testing of blood ammonia requires careful adherence to laboratory protocols to minimize preanalytical variance and spuriously elevated values.
- Historically, ammonia testing has correlated only weakly with the severity of disease in type C HE; however, increasing data point to the prognostic value of ammonia, both in type A and type C HE.

HEPATIC ENCEPHALOPATHY—BACKGROUND

Hepatic encephalopathy (HE) is defined as brain dysfunction caused by liver insufficiency and/or portosystemic shunting, manifesting with a wide array of neurologic and/or psychiatric abnormalities that range from subclinical (or "minimal") alterations to coma.[1] Conditions in which HE occurs include decompensated cirrhosis (type C), acute liver failure (ALF) (type A), and portosystemic shunts (type B), which may be either iatrogenic (eg, surgical shunt or transjugular intrahepatic portosystemic shunt [TIPS]) or an inherent anatomic malformation. HE can be staged using the West Haven Criteria, and more recent updated terminology categorizes HE as either overt (stage 2–4) or covert (minimal to stage 1).

The pathophysiology behind HE is complex and multifactorial. Elevated blood ammonia, a neurotoxin, has long been known to be a necessary component of the syndrome. Ammonia crossing the blood-brain barrier, causing neurologic dysfunction, was thought to be a large part of the pathophysiology dating back over 120 years.

Funding: This work has been supported by an unrestricted grant from The Mark Jordan and Kendall Patton Foundation.
[a] Department of Gastroenterology, California Pacific Medical Center; [b] Division of Hepatology, Department of Advanced Organ Therapies, California Pacific Medical Center
* Corresponding author. 1100 Van Ness Avenue, 3rd Floor, San Francisco, CA 94109,
E-mail address: todd.frederick@sutterhealth.org

Ammonia is produced by the deamination (via glutaminase) of nitrogen-containing amino acids in the intestine (both the microbiome as well as the enterocytes), liver, kidney, brain (astrocytes), and muscle. Conversely, ammonia can be consumed by the reverse process of amination of glutamate (via glutamine synthetase), forming glutamine in these same tissues. The resultant interorgan ammonia trafficking helps to explain the multifactorial nature and flux of hyperammonemia. The elimination of ammonia is achieved via the elimination of nitrogenous wastes, largely via urea (via the hepatocytic urea cycle by way of the kidney) or through the stool, either as a waste product or via bacterial protein synthesis. While the normal functioning liver largely succeeds in maintaining ammonia homeostasis, elevated blood ammonia concentrations can arise due to portosystemic collaterals shunting blood through or around the liver, comorbid renal dysfunction, and sarcopenia leading to decreased ammonia utilization and/or excretion.[1] It is important to keep in mind, however, that an elevated ammonia level, if confirmed, confers a diagnosis of hyperammonemia, which may have other nonhepatic causes. The syndrome of HE appears to require hyperammonemia, but more recent literature points to additional insults that may predispose patients with cirrhosis and portal hypertension to an overt HE event, such as increased permeability of the blood-brain barrier in patients with liver disease, possibly allowing increased NH4 into the central nervous system (CNS); similarly, increased oxidative stress, excess bile acids, and systemic inflammation may play a role in compromising mitochondrial energy production within the brain. Increased ammonia may lead to astrocyte dysfunction due to excess glutamine accumulation (via glutamine synthetase), leading to osmotic swelling, as well as direct mitochondrial toxicity, leading to bioenergetic failure.[2]

The diagnosis of HE is largely a clinical one, without the requirement for any confirmatory laboratory testing in the proper clinical scenario. Laboratory tests, however, can be critical in excluding other diagnoses in conjunction with clinical assessment. Herein, the authors will review the fundamentals of laboratory testing in the evaluation and management of patients suffering from HE.

AMMONIA
Technical Review

Ammonia is an unstable analyte, a byproduct of amino acid metabolism.[3] It exists in both a gaseous form (NH3) and a protonated or ionized form (NH4+). The interchange depends upon the pH of a solution, with more alkaline solutions shifting the balance to more NH3; however, the vast majority of ammonia exists as ammonium (NH4+) at physiologic pH ($\sim$98%). Due to its instability, proper specimen collection and analysis are important for accurate measurement of blood ammonia levels (**Table 1**).

When obtaining a blood ammonia level, either venous or arterial sampling can be used. In theory, the ammonia level in a venous sample would be expected to be lower than in an arterial sample if the muscle, kidney, and brain are contributing to the utilization and disposal of ammonia before venous return. Accordingly, early laboratory investigations demonstrated a significant increase in arterial ammonia compared to simultaneous venous ammonia in a small study of 14 patients with cirrhosis ($P<.01$).[4] However, subsequent studies suggest that arterial levels are similar to venous samples and may not provide additional diagnostic nor prognostic capabilities, particularly in type C HE.[5,6] Other studies, particularly for type A HE in ALF, have suggested the use of arterial ammonia is strongly preferred; however, this was not confirmed in one of the largest retrospective analyses of ammonia in ALF.[5,6] Various society guidelines do not specify the source of the ammonia testing.[1,7,8]

Table 1
Clinical pearls on preanalytical factors associated with ammonia levels

Category	Publication	Outcome
Arterial vs venous source	Snady et al,[4] 1988	Arterial ammonia is significantly greater than venous ammonia (P<.01)
	Nicolao et al,[17] 2003	Arterial, venous, and partial pressure of ammonia were equally limited in their diagnostic and prognostic capabilities.
	Ong et al,[16] 2003	Venous sampling is adequate compared to arterial (r = 0.56 vs 0.61), and there is no advantage of using partial pressure of ammonia (in either venous or arterial samples).
Tourniquet use	Saleem et al,[48] 2009	Tourniquet time of more than 1 min increases hemolysis (OR 19.5, 95% CI 5.6–67.4)
Exercise (or clenched fist) and ammonia levels	Wilkinson et al,[49] 2010	Hyperammonemia occurs in exercise due to increased production from the contracting muscles. Ammonia levels in extreme exercise often surpass those in patients with cirrhosis.
Collection tubes	Goldstein et al,[10] 2017	Lithium heparin tubes were significantly less accurate than EDTA tubes. Lithium tubes may underestimate ammonia levels.
Temperature handling	Nikolac et al,[3] 2014	Samples centrifuged at 0°C had a 9.5% increase in ammonia level compared to 28% increase when centrifuged at room temperature (P=.033). Samples placed in ice immediately after centrifugation had significantly lower increase in ammonia level compared to samples stored at room temperature (13% vs 31%, P=.008)
Timing of specimen processing	Imbert-Bismut et al,[50] 2020	Ammonia samples take longer to arrive to the laboratory through pneumatic tube transport compared to walking the sample to the laboratory. Ammonia concentrations were not affected if the sample is processed within 1.75 h while at 4 °C
	Howanitz et al.[10]	Delay in processing of plasma samples by 24h at 4C increased ammonia levels by 37%
Other analytes may affect ammonia levels	Nikolac et al,[3] 2014	Various serum markers can lead to ammonia bias: ALT: r = 0.38, P = .001; RBC: r = 0.18, P=.025; GGT: r: 0.19, P=.015; WBC: r = 0.178, P=.024.
	da Fonseca-Wollheim,[51] 1990	In vitro formation of ammonia through deamination of glutamine by elevated plasma GGT can increase serum ammonia level by up to 30-fold.
Fasting vs. post-prandial ammonia levels	Bajaj et al,[12] 2020	Cirrhotic patients had a 12% (1h) and 18% (2h) post-prandial increase in ammonia relative to baseline.

Abbreviations: ALT, alanine transaminase; CI, confidence interval; EDTA, ethylenediaminetetraacetic acid; GGT,gamma-glutamyltransferase; OR, odds ratio; RBC, red blood cell; WBC, white blood cell.
Data from Kabara S, R.V., Hepatic Encephalopathy: A Review. European Medical Journal, 2021. 9: p. 89-97.

Additionally, studies have not confirmed the utility of testing the partial pressure of NH3 (representing the nonionized gaseous form) compared to total ammonia (representing gaseous NH3 and ionized NH4). Ultimately, the convenience and safety of venous sampling make this the preferred route for the majority of patients undergoing testing.

Because many factors may influence the ammonia level, it is important to have protocols in place to optimize accuracy in the laboratory measurement of ammonia. Erythrocytes have 3-fold higher concentration of ammonia, so a hemolyzed sample will significantly skew the result. Therefore, free-flowing blood is desired, and a tourniquet should not be used. Additionally, due to the muscle release of ammonia, patients should not clench their hand during blood draw.[3,9] Ethylenediaminetetraacetic acid (lavender top) is the preferred anticoagulant due to concerns of falsely low ammonia levels in the presence of heparin. The specimen tube is ideally pre-chilled and should be filled completely.[10] Since red blood cells are a potential source of ammonia diffusing into the serum, anticoagulated samples should be centrifuged to separate plasma as soon as feasible and ideally within 15 minutes of collection. The importance of promptly separating plasma from red blood cells to avoid spuriously elevated ammonia levels was demonstrated in a study of healthy volunteers noting a near 50% increase between results for heparinized plasma versus whole-blood specimens (30 vs 44 micromol/L, $P < .001$).[11] Following centrifugation, plasma is generally processed as a fresh sample but may also be frozen (−20C or −70C) for up to 24 to 48 hours. Fresh samples are preferred, as frozen samples often report a lower value.[12]

Once properly collected and processed, plasma ammonia can then be measured via either indirect or direct methods. In one indirect method using a point-of-care and dry-slide analyzer, free ammonia is liberated from the sample via alkalization. Ammonia then passes through a semipermeable membrane, changing the color of an ammonium indicator, which is then measured by reflectance spectroscopy. A second and more commonly utilized method directly measures ammonia through its reaction with α-oxo-glutarate and reduced nicotinamide adenine dinucleotide phosphate (NADPH) forming glutamate and NADP+ and water. An absorbance spectrometer can assess NADPH or NADP levels, therefore determining the level of ammonia needed to complete this reaction. A final method also directly measures ammonia concentration using an ammonia avid membrane, which is typically created with a mixture of nonactin and monoactin antibiotics. Ammonia may be reported in conventional units of microgram/dL or in the International System of Units of micromole/L, and it is important to note the difference, with microgram/dL approximately 1.7-fold higher. Conversion calculators are available online.

A pertinent example of how the variability in measurement of ammonia across clinical sites may compromise care can be found in the STOP-HE trial. This randomized clinical trial investigating the use of ornithine phenylacetate for the treatment of overt HE narrowly missed its primary endpoint. A post hoc analysis performed after excluding 30 subjects, initially enrolled with hyperammonemia by local testing but subsequently found to have normal ammonia levels by centralized testing, (an exclusion criterion) appeared to demonstrate a statistically significant benefit for the intervention arm.[13] However, this analysis required retesting of frozen samples which are inherently less reliable than the results from fresh samples.

Diagnostic Capabilities

Given the complex interplay of ammonia and systemic inflammation in the pathophysiology of HE, hyperammonemia by itself cannot confirm a diagnosis of HE; however, it is unusual to diagnose HE in the setting of a normal ammonia level. HE remains a clinical diagnosis; however, an elevated ammonia level may help confirm a diagnosis when there is high pre-test probability of HE diagnosis; and the higher the ammonia the level, the more likely the diagnosis.[14] Patients with decompensated cirrhosis can have a chronically elevated baseline ammonia level with minimal to no signs of encephalopathy; therefore, routine measurement for this population is discouraged. Similar to other analytes commonly measured in clinical practice (ie, ALT), there is no agreed upon value for the upper limit of normal (ULN) of ammonia in the healthy population, nor in the cirrhotic population. Comparison studies across centers have demonstrated significant differences between sites; however, the majority of healthy volunteers demonstrate ammonia levels well below the published ULN.[12] Furthermore, there is no diagnostic threshold for blood ammonia level in diagnosing and managing HE.[1,15] The degree of elevation of ammonia only weakly correlates with severity of symptoms in cirrhosis, presumably due to the synergistic effects of inflammation on the neuropsychiatric effects of ammonia.[2,16] Clinical staging of overt HE, therefore, does not rely upon nor require ammonia measurements but remains the responsibility of the trained clinician.

Contrary to using elevated ammonia levels to diagnose HE, a normal ammonia level can often be used to exclude the diagnosis since the negative predictive value (NPV) of a normal ammonia concentration is high (NPV 0.81).[7,17] The American Association for the Study of Liver Diseases (AASLD) guidance states, "increased blood ammonia alone does not add any diagnostic, staging, or prognostic value for HE in patients with chronic liver disease. A normal value calls for diagnostic re-evaluation (GRADE II-3, A, 1)."[1] Additionally, more recently updated guidance from the European Association for the Study of the Liver (EASL) also recommends plasma ammonia testing primarily for its NPV in patients with cirrhosis.[8]

Clinicians less experienced in the diagnosis and management of overt HE may find the measurement of ammonia useful for confirming clinical suspicion, but routine measurement of ammonia for patients with cirrhosis presenting without an altered sensorium should be discouraged.[18] Studies observing trends in ordering blood ammonia have found that nearly a third of clinicians recommend routine ammonia testing in patients with grade 2 to 4 overt HE; however, of note, significantly fewer trainee physicians are likely to do so.[19] Current national trends suggest that practitioners are ordering ammonia testing at increasing rates for patients with compensated cirrhosis, quadrupling from 1.3 to 5.7 tests per 1000 inpatient days in 2007 to 2015 (P=.017); and a less pronounced increase for those with decompensated cirrhosis, rising from 7.7 to 13.1 tests per 1000 inpatient days.[20] This increase was postulated to be due to implementation of the electronic medical record and ability to routinely order these tests. However, despite the increases, the overall rates of ammonia testing appear to be low, representing only 1.9% and 4.5% of total hospitalizations in compensated and decompensated cirrhotic patients, respectively.[20] Finally, when clinicians do order ammonia levels in patients with HE, it often does not change management as 1 single-center study retrospectively examining total lactulose dosing determined. The investigators analyzed over 1200 patient admissions for HE, including 46% with the measurement of ammonia, and found that overall lactulose dosing did not differ between the groups.[15]

Prognostic Value

While ammonia cannot be used alone to diagnose HE, there is a growing literature supporting measurement of ammonia as a prognostic factor. This has been well established in patients with ALF.[5,21–23] Similarly, reduction in ammonia is associated with better outcomes in patients with ALF.[24,25] However, utilizing ammonia for prognosis in patients with chronic liver disease has been considered controversial. Evidence now exists to challenge the AASLD guidance statement dismissing the prognostic value of ammonia for the diagnosis of HE.

In a large multicenter study of 726 stable outpatients with cirrhosis, investigators found a compelling increased risk of both hospitalization and mortality for patients with elevated ammonia (hazard ratio [HR] 2.13, confidence interval [CI] 1.89–2.40, $P<.001$; HR 1.45, CI 1.2–1.76, $P<.001$, respectively).[26] A cutoff of 1.4x the local ULN best predicted risk. It is important to note that both arterial and venous samples were utilized but were collected under a careful protocol at each site utilizing chilled collection tubes and rapid processing. The investigators also minimized variability across sites by utilizing internal controls at each laboratory and transforming each patient value to a multiple of the local ULN (termed AMM-ULN in the article).[26] For patients with documented HE, there are conflicting reports whether ammonia levels correlate with the severity of HE.[16,17] Other studies have found that ammonia can be an independent predictor of 28-day mortality and a lack of improvement to baseline ammonia by hospital day 5 is associated with high mortality.[27]

Another compelling example of the predictive capability of outpatient ammonia monitoring came from a retrospective analysis of the randomized controlled trial evaluating the ammonia scavenger, glycerol phenylbutyrate, for the prevention of HE.[28,29] The investigators collected fasting venous blood samples at baseline and days 7 and 14 of the 16-week trial. Ammonia levels were categorized in relation to the standardized ULN as follows: less than 1.0 x ULN, greater than 1.0 x ULN, less than 1.5 x ULN, greater than 1.5 x ULN. Patients with ammonia levels in the highest category (>1.5 x ULN) developed overt HE episodes at twice the rate of those with lower ammonia levels ($P = .002$).

OTHER LABORATORY TESTING IN HEPATIC ENCEPHALOPATHY

When making a diagnosis of HE, it is important to consider a broad differential diagnosis and appropriately exclude other potential etiologies for altered mental status. Various laboratory tests to be considered can be found in **Table 2**. Additional

Table 2 Laboratory testing beyond ammonia for the evaluation of altered mentation in patients with cirrhosis	
Higher yield	• Comprehensive metabolic panel including calcium, magnesium, and phosphate • Complete blood count • Thyroid-stimulating hormone (TSH) • Blood culture • Urinalysis with reflex to urine culture • Urine and/or blood toxicology screen • Blood alcohol level • Lactic acid
Lower yield	• Sedimentation rate (ESR) • C-reactive protein (CRP) • Thiamine • Vitamin B12 • Human immunodeficiency virus serology • Syphilis serology • Cerebrospinal fluid analysis (required if meningismus present)

considerations for laboratory testing in the diagnosis and management of HE are outlined in the following sections.

Thyroid Axis

Hypothyroidism is believed to cause hyperammonemia through the downregulation of ammonia metabolism to urea and possibly through concomitant myopathy.[30–33] In a multicenter prospective analysis (NACSELD-2), low thyroxine (as well as low maltose, high methyl-4-hydroxybenzoate sulfate, and high 3,4-dihydroxybutyrate) levels predicted advanced HE development.[34] In multivariable logistic regression analysis, thyroxine levels were an independent predictor of advanced HE (OR 0.67, CI 0.48–0.89, $P = .01$). Similarly, in a single-center prospective cohort study of 122 patients with hepatitis B virus (HBV)–related acute-on-chronic liver failure (ACLF), free triiodothyronine (FT3) level, and its change over time enhanced prediction of 90-day prognosis, with an area under the receiver operating characteristic curve of 0.892.[35]

Interleukin–6

Interleukin-6 (IL-6) is an important cytokine driving systemic inflammation, and its presence has been associated with both covert and overt HE. IL-6 serum levels may help diagnose minimal HE (MHE), as levels $\geq$ 8pg/mL discriminated against patients with and without MHE with a receiver operating characteristic of 0.751, whereas a level $\geq$ 7pg/mL had a sensitivity of 90% with an NPV of 93%.[36] Another study assessing risks of overt HE following TIPS, found a pre-procedure serum IL-6 level greater than 10.5 pg/mL predicted post-TIPS overt HE with an area under the curve (AUC) of 0.83.[37] IL-6 was an independent risk factor for overall overt HE (RR = 1.154, $P<.001$) and for stage 4 HE (coma) (RR 1.051, $P=.019$).[37] Similarly, in a study evaluating predictors of future overt HE, patients with an IL-6 above the median of 9 pg/mL developed overt HE much more often (35.6% vs 1.9, $P<.001$).[38] In a subset of patients without prior overt HE, the predictive performance of IL-6 was better than the model for end-stage liver disease (MELD) (AUC 0.966 vs 0.843) with the ideal cut off for IL-6 of 23.5 pg/mL, with sensitivity and specificity of 89.3% and 89.5%, respectively.[38]

Endotoxin and the Microbiome

The microbiome has been implicated in the pathogenesis of HE through the release of endotoxin as well as both increased intestinal ammonia release (via urease) and absorption (incorporated into amino acid and protein production). Endotoxemia is thought to occur in the setting of both intestinal dysbiosis and an impaired intestinal epithelial barrier ("leaky gut"). Studies have found that patients with liver disease have reduced variation in microbial species. This reduction in species diversity is even more pronounced in patients with HE.[39] One study found 8 fecal bacterial species were associated with overt HE, although these species could not predict future overt HE.[40] Endotoxin, or lipopolysaccharide, is released by gram-negative bacteria and induces an inflammatory cascade upon absorption into the liver via activation of Kupffer cells. Studies have found that patients with cirrhosis and HE often have elevated serum endotoxin levels compared to patients with cirrhosis without HE (0.27 $\pm$ 0.24, 0.059 $\pm$ 0.012, respectively, $P=.002$).[41] Short-chain fatty acids, products of bacterial metabolism, have also been implicated in HE, although studies are conflicting, and this association has not been well established. While 1 study found overt HE associated with lower levels of certain short-chain fatty acids, another study found no association.[39,40] Other investigators have utilized machine learning to create prediction models for the development of HE based upon oral or fecal microbiota, finding fecal microbiota had superior discrimination ability when identifying patients with cirrhosis with or without overt HE by history.[42]

OTHER EXPERIMENTAL LABORATORY WORKS

Interest in alternative means of measuring ammonia has led to ammonia breath testing. In 1 study, an elevated vaporized ammonia level of $\geq$165 ppb had an AUC of 0.86 in distinguishing between patients with cirrhosis versus healthy controls (95% CI: 0.79–0.93), and a breath ammonia level $\geq$ 175 ppb could distinguish between cirrhotic patients with and without HE with an AUC of 0.83 (95% CI: 0.73–0.94).[43] This may be an avenue for future research, especially as a potential point-of-care test in the outpatient setting. A recent proof-of-concept publication of a product called Wize Sniffer, an electronic semiconductor gas sensor, found that TGS2602, which detects ammonia, hydrogen sulfide, ethanol, and hydrogen, had an AUC of 0.864 (95% CI 0.662–1, P = .00) in differentiating between cirrhosis with and without HE at a value of 0.065.[44]

Microbially derived metabolites have been found to be associated with overt HE.[34] In 1 multicenter inpatient cohort, high methyl-4-hydroxybenzoate sulfate and 3,4-dihydroxybutyrate levels, both bacterial metabolites, along with low thyroxine, lysophospholipids, and isoleucine, were associated with overt HE with an AUC 0.87 to 0.9. Other studies investigating metabolites have found that in comparing patients with hepatitis B cirrhosis with MHE versus no HE, 27 small-molecule metabolites were found to be potential biomarkers for MHE[45]

Research focused on the CNS has observed that biomarkers of various neurons may be implicated in HE. Glial fibrillary acidic protein (GFAP) elevation in the serum is a marker of astrocyte injury. Gairing and colleagues[46] found that serum GFAP was elevated in cirrhotic patients with covert HE compared to those without (median GFAP 163pg/ml [interquartile range (IQR) 136;268] vs 106 pg/mL [IQR 75;153, P<.001). However, not all neurologic metabolites are diagnostically helpful. Serum S100 B is expressed in astrocytes and other glial cells. One study found S100 B to be less effective than ammonia in diagnosing covert HE.[47]

SUMMARY

Laboratory testing for the diagnosis and management of HE is largely focused on identifying possible precipitating factors and excluding other conditions. HE remains both a clinical diagnosis and one of exclusion. The nature and extent of laboratory testing will vary according to clinical circumstances. The testing of ammonia levels in the blood can be helpful when the diagnosis is in question but is neither required for confirmation in the proper clinical context nor is ammonia testing necessary for staging or prognosis with a few key exceptions: ALF, and possibly ACLF, where it can correlate with intracranial hypertension and mortality risk. Monitoring of the patient receiving treatment for HE does not require repeated ammonia testing unless the diagnosis is called into question or if treating patients with known or suspected intracranial hypertension. An argument can also be made to follow blood ammonia levels when treating patients with therapies specifically targeted at reducing hyperammonemia. More recent literature is lending support to the prognostic capabilities inherent in ammonia levels in the blood of cirrhotic patients, both in predicting future HE events and in determining outcomes in hospitalized patients. If ammonia levels are to be tested and relied upon, one must have strict protocols in place to control preanalytical factors and collection methods to avoid common pitfalls in the measurement of this labile analyte. Newer and novel biomarkers are being explored for the diagnosis and management of HE, including IL-6 and other inflammatory markers, and results are encouraging. Further studies investigating the utility of other laboratory-based testing to diagnose, stage, or predict HE, including evaluating severity of systemic inflammation, fecal microbiota, bacterial metabolites, and neurologic biomarkers are encouraged.

CLINICS CARE POINTS

- Ammonia remains key to the pathophysiology of hepatic encephalopathy
- False elevations of ammonia occur with delays in centrifugation and processing, storing blood at room temperature, utilizing a tourniquet and/or clenching fist for blood draw, and in patients with significantly elevated ALT and/or GGT given their intrinsic enzymatic acitivites
- Ammonia tends to be higher in arterial and post-prandial blood samples

DISCLOSURE

R.T. Frederick serves as an investigator for Salix Pharmaceuticals/Bausch Health, Mallinckrodt, Astra Zeneca, River 2 Renal; a consultant for Mallinckrodt, Seal Rock Therapeutics, Tennor Therapeutics.

REFERENCES

1. Vilstrup H, Amodio P, Bajaj J, et al. Hepatic encephalopathy in chronic liver disease: 2014 practice guideline by the American association for the study of liver diseases and the European association for the study of the liver. Hepatology 2014;60(2):715–35.
2. Rose CF, Amodio P, Bajaj JS, et al. Hepatic encephalopathy: novel insights into classification, pathophysiology and therapy. J Hepatol 2020;73(6):1526–47.
3. Nikolac N, Omazic J, Simundic AM. The evidence based practice for optimal sample quality for ammonia measurement. Clin Biochem 2014;47(12):991–5.
4. Snady H, Lieber CS. Venous, arterial, and arterialized-venous blood ammonia levels and their relationship to hepatic encephalopathy after propranolol. Am J Gastroenterol 1988;83(3):249–55.
5. Cardoso FS, Gottfried M, Tujios S, et al. US Acute Liver Failure Study Group. Continuous renal replacement therapy is associated with reduced serum ammonia levels and mortality in acute liver failure. Hepatology 2018;67(2):711–20.
6. Kalal C, Shukla A, Mohanka R, et al. Should venous ammonia be used in decision-making acute liver failure patients? Hepatology 2018;67(2):800–1.
7. Drolz A, Jäger B, Wewalka M, et al. Clinical impact of arterial ammonia levels in ICU patients with different liver diseases. Intensive Care Med 2013;39(7):1227–37.
8. Montagnese S, Rautou PE, Romero-Gómez M, et al. EASL Clinical Practice Guidelines on the management of hepatic encephalopathy. J Hepatol 2022;77(3):807–24.
9. Lowenstein JM. Ammonia production in muscle and other tissues: the purine nucleotide cycle. Physiol Rev 1972;52(2):382–414.
10. Goldstein BN, Wesler J, Nowacki AS, et al. Investigations of blood ammonia analysis: test matrices, storage, and stability. Clin Biochem 2017;50(9):537–9.
11. Howanitz JH, Howanitz PJ, Skrodzki CA, et al. Influences of specimen processing and storage conditions on results for plasma ammonia. Clin Chem 1984;30(6):906–8.

12. Bajaj JS, Bloom PP, Chung RT, et al. Variability and lability of ammonia levels in healthy volunteers and patients with cirrhosis: Implications for trial design and clinical practice. Am J Gastroenterol 2020;115(5):783–5.
13. Rahimi RS, Safadi R, Thabut D, et al. Efficacy and safety of ornithine phenylacetate for treating overt hepatic encephalopathy in a randomized trial. Clin Gastroenterol Hepatol 2021;19(12):2626–35.e7.
14. Deutsch-Link S, Moon AM. The Ongoing Debate of serum ammonia levels in cirrhosis: the Good, the Bad, and the Ugly. Am J Gastroenterol 2023;118(1):10–3.
15. Haj M, Rockey DC. Ammonia levels do not guide clinical management of patients with hepatic encephalopathy caused by cirrhosis. Am J Gastroenterol 2020; 115(5):723–8.
16. Ong JP, Aggarwal A, Krieger D, et al. Correlation between ammonia levels and the severity of hepatic encephalopathy. Am J Med 2003;114(3):188–93.
17. Nicolao F, Efrati C, Masini A, et al. Role of determination of partial pressure of ammonia in cirrhotic patients with and without hepatic encephalopathy. J Hepatol 2003;38(4):441–6.
18. Tapper EB, Jiang ZG, Patwardhan VR. Refining the ammonia hypothesis: a physiology-driven approach to the treatment of hepatic encephalopathy. Mayo Clin Proc 2015;90(5):646–58.
19. Reuter B, Walter K, Bissonnette J, et al. Assessment of the spectrum of hepatic encephalopathy: a multicenter study. Liver Transpl 2018;24(5):587–94.
20. Deutsch-Link S, Moon AM, Jiang Y, et al. Serum ammonia in cirrhosis: clinical impact of hyperammonemia, utility of testing, and national testing trends. Clin Ther 2022;44(3):e45–57.
21. Clemmesen JO, Larsen FS, Kondrup J, et al. Cerebral herniation in patients with acute E liver failure is correlated with arterial ammonia concentration. Hepatology 1999;29(3):648–53.
22. Kundra A, Jain A, Banga A, et al. Evaluation of plasma ammonia levels in patients with acute liver failure and chronic liver disease and its correlation with the severity of hepatic encephalopathy and clinical features of raised intracranial tension. Clin Biochem 2005;38(8):696–9.
23. Bernal W, Hall C, Karvellas CJ, et al. Arterial ammonia and clinical risk factors for encephalopathy and intracranial hypertension in acute liver failure. Hepatology 2007;46(6):1844–52.
24. Niranjan-Azadi AM, Araz F, Patel YA, et al. Ammonia level and mortality in acute liver failure: a single-center experience. Ann Transplant 2016;21:479–83.
25. Bhatia V. Predictive value of arterial ammonia for complications and outcome in acute liver failure. Gut 2006;55(1):98–104.
26. Tranah TH, Ballester MP, Carbonell-Asins JA, et al. Plasma ammonia levels predict hospitalisation with liver-related complications and mortality in clinically stable outpatients with cirrhosis. J Hepatol 2022;77(6):1554–63.
27. Shalimar, Sheikh MF, Mookerjee RP, et al. Prognostic role of ammonia in patients with cirrhosis. Hepatology 2019;70(3):982–94.
28. Vierling JM, Mokhtarani M, Brown RS, et al. Fasting blood ammonia predicts risk and Frequency of hepatic encephalopathy episodes in patients with cirrhosis. Clin Gastroenterol Hepatol 2016;14(6):903–6.e1.
29. Rockey DC, Vierling JM, Mantry P, et al. Randomized, double-blind, controlled study of glycerol phenylbutyrate in hepatic encephalopathy. Hepatology 2014; 59(3):1073–83.
30. Rimar D, Kruzel-Davila E, Dori G, et al. Hyperammonemic coma—Barking up the Wrong tree. J Gen Intern Med 2007;22(4):549–52.

31. Thobe N, Pilger P, Jones MP. Primary hypothyroidism masquerading as hepatic encephalopathy: case report and review of the literature. Postgrad Med J 2000;76(897):424–6.
32. Díaz-Fontenla F, Castillo-Pradillo M, Díaz-Gómez A, et al. Refractory hepatic encephalopathy in a patient with hypothyroidism: another element in ammonia metabolism. World J Gastroenterol 2017;23(28):5246.
33. Diaz-Fontenla F, Castillo M, Díaz-Gomez A, et al. Refractory hepatic encephalopathy and hypothyroidism: a New factor in the ammonia metabolism. J Clin Exp Hepatol 2017;7:S47–9.
34. Bajaj JS, Tandon P, O'Leary JG, et al. Admission serum metabolites and thyroxine predict advanced hepatic encephalopathy in a multicenter inpatient cirrhosis cohort. Clin Gastroenterol Hepatol 2022. https://doi.org/10.1016/j.cgh.2022.03.046.
35. Zhang J, Chen Y, Ding M, et al. Correlation between dynamic changes in free triiodothyronine levels and 90-day prognosis in patients with HBV-related acute-on-chronic liver failure. Eur J Med Res 2022;27(1). https://doi.org/10.1186/s40001-022-00718-8.
36. Gairing SJ, Anders J, Kaps L, et al. Evaluation of IL-6 for Stepwise diagnosis of minimal hepatic encephalopathy in patients with liver cirrhosis. Hepatol Commun 2021;6(5):2022.
37. Li J, Liu Y, Li M, et al. Association of preoperative IL-6 levels with overt HE in patients with cirrhosis after TIPS. Hepatol Commun 2023;7(4). https://doi.org/10.1097/HC9.0000000000000128.
38. Labenz C, Toenges G, Huber Y, et al. Raised serum Interleukin-6 identifies patients with liver cirrhosis at high risk for overt hepatic encephalopathy. Aliment Pharmacol Ther 2019;50(10):1112–9.
39. Wang Q, Chen C, Zuo S, et al. Integrative analysis of the gut microbiota and faecal and serum short-chain fatty acids and tryptophan metabolites in patients with cirrhosis and hepatic encephalopathy. J Transl Med 2023;21(1):395.
40. Bloom PP, Luévano JM, Miller KJ, et al. Deep stool microbiome analysis in cirrhosis reveals an association between short-chain fatty acids and hepatic encephalopathy. Ann Hepatol 2021;25:100333.
41. Bajaj JS, Ridlon JM, Hylemon PB, et al. Linkage of gut microbiome with cognition in hepatic encephalopathy. Am J Physiol Gastrointest Liver Physiol 2012;302(1):G168–75.
42. Saboo K, Petrakov NV, Shamsaddini A, et al. Stool microbiota are superior to saliva in distinguishing cirrhosis and hepatic encephalopathy using machine learning. J Hepatol 2022;76(3):600–7.
43. Adrover R, Cocozzella D, Ridruejo E, et al. Breath-ammonia testing of healthy subjects and patients with cirrhosis. Dig Dis Sci 2012;57(1):189–95.
44. Germanese D, Colantonio S, D'Acunto M, et al. An E-Nose for the monitoring of Severe liver Impairment: a Preliminary study. Sensors (Basel) 2019;19(17). https://doi.org/10.3390/s19173656.
45. Huang G, Xie S, Wang M, et al. Metabolite profiling analysis of hepatitis B virus–induced liver cirrhosis patients with minimal hepatic encephalopathy using gas chromatography-time-of-flight mass spectrometry and ultra-performance liquid chromatography-quadrupole-time-of-flight mass spectrometry. Biomed Chromatogr 2023;37(1). https://doi.org/10.1002/bmc.5529.
46. Gairing SJ, Danneberg S, Kaps L, et al. Elevated serum levels of glial fibrillary acidic protein are associated with covert hepatic encephalopathy in patients with cirrhosis. JHEP Reports 2023;5(4):100671.

47. Kim MJ, Kim JH, Jung JH, et al. Serum S100B levels in patients with liver cirrhosis and hepatic encephalopathy. Diagnostics 2023;13(3). https://doi.org/10.3390/diagnostics13030333.

48. Saleem S, Mani V, Chadwick MA, et al. A prospective study of causes of haemolysis during venepuncture: tourniquet time should be kept to a minimum. Ann Clin Biochem Int J Lab Med 2009;46(3):244–6.

49. Wilkinson DJ, Smeeton NJ, Watt PW. Ammonia metabolism, the brain and fatigue; revisiting the link. Prog Neurobiol 2010;91(3):200–19.

50. Imbert-Bismut F, Payet PE, Alfaisal J, et al. Transportation and handling of blood samples prior to ammonia measurement in the real life of a large university hospital. Clin Chim Acta 2020;510:522–30.

51. da Fonseca-Wollheim F. Deamidation of glutamine by increased plasma gamma-glutamyltransferase is a source of rapid ammonia formation in blood and plasma specimens. Clin Chem 1990;36(8 Pt 1):1479–82.

Minimal Hepatic Encephalopathy

Rachel Redfield, MD[a], Nyan Latt, MD[b], Santiago J. Munoz, MD[c],*

KEYWORDS

- Encephalopathy • Ammonia • Cirrhosis • Minimal • Covert • Cognitive • Attention
- Confusion

KEY POINTS

- Minimal hepatic encephalopathy (MHE) is a frequent complication of cirrhosis characterized by subtle mental dysfunction.
- MHE nonetheless causes diminished quality of life and impairs driving motor vehicles to a variable extent.
- Smartphone applications such as EncephalApp-Stroop test are able to detect attention and cognitive defects associated with MHE.
- Therapy with lactulose can improve the psychometric abnormalities of MHE but the therapy can cause gastrointestinal symptoms such as diarrhea, flatulence, and abdominal discomfort.
- More research is needed to determine when and how MHE should be treated.

INTRODUCTION

Minimal hepatic encephalopathy (MHE) affects a large proportion of patients with cirrhosis, has demonstrated real and important consequences and impact on daily life, including impaired driving performance, increased vehicle accidents and traffic violations, diminished quality of life, unemployment, and propensity to falls, and predicts transition to overt HE, namely, decompensation of the cirrhosis (**Box 1**).

Given the absence of specific signs or symptoms associated with MHE, the study of its natural history has been particularly challenging and remains minimally understood. At present, it is clear that a significant proportion of patients with MHE go on to eventually develop overt hepatic encephalopathy (OHE). Known risk factors for such progression include male gender, prior history of OHE, alcohol etiology of the cirrhosis,

[a] Thomas Jefferson Hospital, Division of Gastroenterology, 132 S. 10th Street, Suite 480, Philadelphia, PA 19106, USA; [b] Virtua Health System, Center for Liver Disease and Transplant Program, 63 Kresson Road, Suite 101, Cherry Hill, NJ 08034, USA; [c] The Johns Hopkins University School of Medicine and Medical Institutions, Division of Gastroenterology and Hepatology, 600 N. Wolfe Street, Blalock Building, Suite 465, Baltimore, MD 21287, USA
* Corresponding author. 600 N. Wolfe Street, Blalock 465, Baltimore, MD 21287.
E-mail address: Smunoz2@jhmi.edu

Clin Liver Dis 28 (2024) 237–252
https://doi.org/10.1016/j.cld.2024.01.004
1089-3261/24/© 2024 Elsevier Inc. All rights reserved.

Box 1
Impact of minimal hepatic encephalopathy[a,b]

Impaired ability to drive motor vehicles

Increased risk of traffic accidents

Impaired ability to operate machinery

Impaired performance and fitness to work

Decreased quality of life (HRQOL)

Increased risk of falls

Decreased home management skills

Difficulties with emotional behavior

Worse sleep quality

[a]Note that not all the above consequences are present in every patient with MHE as its impact can markedly vary in individual patients. [b]Financial impact of MHE on patient and society has not yet been estimated.

---

and those with esophagogastric varices. Likely but yet unproven factors affecting the natural history of MHE and progression to OHE include raising model for end stage liver disease (MELD) score, worsening of the underlying liver disease (eg, having a progressive and/or intractable etiology of the underlying cirrhosis such as metabolic-associated fatty liver disease, autoimmune liver disease resistant to current therapies, alcohol-associated cirrhosis with continued alcohol, and drinking), and onset of decompensation. However, more granular information on the natural history of MHE is not available, and several critical questions remain unanswered. Such questions include (1) whether MHE evolves with exacerbations and flares alternating with periods of remission? (2) what are the precipitating factors that temporarily worsen MHE? (3) are there significant interactions of MHE with concomitant neuropsychiatric entities such as depression, bipolar, substance use disorders, or the natural cognitive decline of aging? (4) is there potential modulation of MHE severity and evolution by environmental factors? (5) does MHE lead to irreversible subclinical cognitive deficits? and (6) is liver transplantation able to reverse the psychometric abnormalities of MHE? The answers to these and other equally relevant questions characterizing the natural history of MHE await clinical research that requires following up the MHE diagnostic tools over time while evaluating effect on outcomes by the above factors. Given the uncertainties about the natural history of MHE, it is suggested and seems reasonable to screen for MHE patients with cirrhosis every 6 to 12 months to be able to detect MHE and go over the need (or not) for therapeutic intervention.

The absence of verbal deficits, confusion, disorientation, and asterixis in MHE results in a patient who appears and performs well in the office visit. Thus, the diagnosis of MHE is currently only possible by performing specialized psychometric and neurophysiological testing, not fitted for routine clinical practice. The term "minimal" is misleading because of the effects of MHE on patients are not trivial. MHE is currently considered the earliest form of "covert" HE. Covert HE includes MHE but also stage I HE which may have already clinically detectable but subtle cognitive deficits (yet no asterixis, a marker of stage II overt HE), which may also be difficult to diagnose in a busy hepatology practice. Thus, the diagnosis of MHE still rests primarily on the ability to perform specialized testing, which fortunately has been gradually refined and shortened, getting closer to routine applicability in the office setting. Given the high frequency of MHE in cirrhosis and its consequences, ideally all patients with cirrhosis should undergo screening tests for MHE. However, this is not yet pragmatic and the current guidelines suggest a focused approach, with MHE testing pursued in patients with cirrhosis who report employment difficulties, nonspecific neurologic symptoms, traffic violations, and motor vehicle accidents. The authors review the most commonly used tests to identify MHE, their performance, and limitation as follows.

ASSESSMENT OF MINIMAL HEPATIC ENCEPHALOPATHY

The compilation of cognitive deficits found in MHE, known as SONIC (spectrum of neurocognitive impairment in cirrhosis), includes changes in attention, working memory, response inhibition, and executive function.[1] Performing specialized neuropsychiatric tests have been the traditional approach to diagnose these subtle cognitive disturbances.[1,2] However, many of these tests are time-consuming, costly, and cannot realistically be implemented in clinical practice by providers taking care of a complex chronic diseases such as cirrhosis. The role of these tests is primarily for research purposes as the gold standard, and therefore, providers should be familiar with them.[3]

Patients with MHE are known to have poorer quality of life as well as risk of falls, impaired driving, and potentially danger operating heavy machinery.[4–6] For this reason, it is important for a hepatology practice to implement routine diagnostic tools to better identify those patients experiencing MHE. In addition, patients with MHE are at high risk for transitioning to overt HE, considered one of the events that defines decompensation in cirrhosis.[7] Traditionally thought to be reversible, there is emerging evidence that patients with a history of overt HE have persistent cognitive dysfunction even post-liver transplantation.[8] As care for chronic liver disease patients shifts toward prevention of first decompensation event (overt HE, variceal bleed, ascites), it has become increasingly important to identify patients who may be at high risk for development of overt encephalopathy.[9] Patients with cirrhosis and MHE are at risk for developing overt HE over time. Furthermore, there is an increased use of transjugular intrahepatic portosystemic shunt (TIPS) for its transplant-free survival benefit, but additional research is required to determine if pre-TIPS MHE is a risk factor for development of post-TIPS overt HE.[10]

Potentially primary prevention of overt HE will soon become standard of care. To do this, we need to understand the diagnostic tools available to diagnose MHE before the onset of overt HE. General intake questions include screening for sleep disturbances, falls, and irritability. These symptoms are more easily reported with recall by patients. Assessing for executive function, psychomotor speed, response inhibition, and working memory deficits require more invasive testing rather than self-assessment (**Box 2**).[11]

The most recent AASLD practice guidelines regarding diagnosis of MHE, published in 2014, recommend that every patient with chronic liver disease be tested for minimal (or covert) HE.[7] A consensus by the International Society for Hepatic Encephalopathy and Nitrogen Metabolism reviewed the testing strategies for covert/minimal HE and discouraged the use of more than one test to diagnose minimal/covert HE to prevent excluding patients who may benefit from counseling or treatment.[12] This consensus also suggested that until there is broad validation of tests, diagnostic tools for MHE can be used after initial screening or self-reported symptoms raise concern. The authors agree that all patients with cirrhosis should be screened for MHE due to the MHE consequences outlined above. Furthermore, early diagnosis of MHE is important to improve quality of life and to identify patients who are at risk of developing OHE and decompensated cirrhosis. **Box 3** summarize the strengths and limitations of some of the commonly used tests to diagnoses MHE.

Box 2
Assessment and diagnostic tests for minimal hepatic encephalopathy

Psychometric Hepatic Encephalopathy Score (PHES):
- Number connection test A and B
- Digital symbol test
- Line tracing test
- Serial dotting test

Inhibitory Control Test (ICT)

Smartphone Applications
- EncephalApp-Stroop Test
- QuickStroop

Animal Naming Tests
- ANT_1
- $S-ANT_1$

Predictors of Onset of Overt Hepatic Encephalopathy
- BABS
- MASQ: HE

PEN AND PAPER TESTS

The most frequently published test and considered the gold standard for identifying minimal cognitive dysfunction in chronic liver disease is the Psychometric Hepatic Encephalopathy Scores (PHESs), which is a series of five paper and pencil tests and is

---

Box 3
Strengths and limitations of tests used in the diagnosis of minimal hepatic encephalopathy

Test	Strengths	Limitations
PHES	Considered gold standard Simple to administer Predicts OHE and survival Validated	Insensitive to early changes Expensive; copyrighted Influenced by age and educational level Learning effect
Inhibitory Control Test	Rapid, less expensive Extensive validation	Requires patient's familiarity with computers Requires high functional level
EEG	Validated for stage I covert HE	Requires specialized equipment; nonspecific
Smart Phone Stroop App Test	Rapid, simple, sensitive Validated, smart phone App	Influenced by age and educational level Training effect
SIP-CHE (Short Version)	High sensitivity, lower specificity Potentially suitable for office/POC use Able to predict onset of OHE Applicable to covert HE	Learning effect on repeat testing Calculators not yet readily available
Animal Naming Test	Rapid (1 minute to complete) Inexpensive, apt for office use Correlated with future OHE Associated also with frailty and disability	Requires further validation in MHE Influenced by age and educational level

Abbreviation: PHESs, Psychometric Hepatic Encephalopathy Scores; POC, point of care.[2,13]

validated in several countries. PHES includes number connection test A (NCT-A), number connection test B (NCT-B), digit symbol test, line tracing test, and serial dotting test.[2] This series takes at least 15 minutes to complete and should ideally be administered and interpreted by a trained clinician. Although the PHES is not routinely used in clinical practice, it is important to be familiar with this battery of pen and paper tests as it is often used in publications to study MHE and validate newer diagnostic tools.[13]

Initial Screening for Minimal Hepatic Encephalopathy

Sickness impact profile covert hepatic encephalopathy

The importance of screening and diagnosing patients with MHE is that development of MHE significantly impacts health-related quality of life (HRQOL).[14] The Sickness Impact Profile (SIP) is a 136-statement questionnaire measuring quality of life but difficult to realistically use in hepatology clinical practice due to its length.[14] A proposed shortened version (SIP covert hepatic encephalopathy, SIP CHE) was developed by Nabi and colleagues to be readily integrated into a busy hepatology practice and includes four of the statements from SIP while also considering sex and age.[15] Of note, the patient population studied did not have history of overt encephalopathy and included diverse etiologies of cirrhosis. The SIP covert hepatic encephalopathy (CHE) is not a test of cognition but could identify MHE with a sensitivity and specificity of 80% and 79%, respectively. Of note, the specificity of SIP CHE decreased on repeat testing at 6 and 12 months.[15]

SIP CHE = −0.6 + 0.1*Age+0.9*male gender+2.6*BCM4+2.4*EB7+1.9*RP8+1.9*E1

BCM4: "I do not maintain balance"
EB7: "I act irritable or impatient with myself"
RP8: "I am not doing any of my usual physical recreation or activities"
E1: "I am eating much less than usual"
SIP CHE was then validated in 2020 with a Danish cross-sectional study of 110 outpatients and also used to determine future development of overt HE.[14] The study used continuous reaction time computerized test and PHES as the gold standard for diagnosing MHE and found that SIP CHE had a high sensitivity (82%) but a relatively low specificity at 38%.[14] The patients were then followed for an average of 2.7 years, during which time SIP CHE had an 87% sensitivity for predicting future development of overt HE. Currently, there are no readily accessible calculators to use the SIP CHE score in clinical practice/point of care. Thus, a suggested area of research is to evaluate the compliance and performance of SIP CHE calculator incorporation into current electronic medical record (EMR) systems.

Computerized Tests at the Point of Care

Point of care tests have become the most clinically relevant ways of diagnosing MHE in office.[11] The creation of cell phone and tablet applications has also improved availability and makes in-office evaluation and diagnosis more feasible.

Inhibitory control test

The inhibitory control test (ICT) is a computer-based test that takes 15 minutes to administer to assess attention and response inhibition.[16,17] This is a computer-based test where the patient is exposed to flashing letters. Participants are instructed to press the spacebar after seeing the "target" which is when the letter Y follows the letter X or vice-versa. There are times where an X follows an X and Y follows a Y, called "lures." The software measures the response and reaction time for both targets and lures. High lure and low target response indicates poorer score and, in the appropriate setting (cirrhosis), MHE.

The ICT was validated in the United States by Bajaj and colleagues using a cutoff of $\geq$5 lures per person to diagnose MHE with a sensitivity of 88% and a specificity of 77%.[16] A battery of pen and pencil tests and block design test (BDT) was used as the gold standard to diagnose MHE in this cohort. The ICT test does not require trained psychologist or personnel to administer but requires the computer program to be downloaded. In addition, ICT requires patients to be comfortable with computer-based tests and takes longer to administer than other point of care tests discussed above.[18]

The smartphone application EncephalApp-Stroop test

The Stroop test is often used in attention-deficit disorders and cognitive impairment to assess psychomotor speed, attention, and impulse inhibition (executive function).[19] Impaired attention and cognitive functions are the hallmark abnormalities found in MHE. These deficits can be detected via assessment of response to auditory trigger events or Stroop-based tasks.[20] A free smart phone and tablet version (EncephalApp-Stroop) was developed making this a nearly ideal point of care tool to use in the assessment of MHE.[21,22]

The EncephalApp-Stroop test also does not need a trained clinician to interpret the results and can be completed before clinic visits or at home in less than 5 minutes. There are five runs in the "Off state" followed by five runs in the "On state." In the "Off state," the Stroop test requires patients to focus on visually presented stimulus (hashtag) to determine its color and then respond with a timed motor action (clicking the correct color). The second part of the Stroop test, "On state," requires attention on the words red, blue, and green which are presented in incongruent colors. For example, the word "red" will be written in a green color. Patients must correctly identify the color of the letters and not the color of the letters that is spelled. The total time in seconds to complete five series correctly is recorded.

The US-based multicenter study by Allampati and colleagues validated the EncephalApp-Stroop tests using two gold standards, PHES (score $\leq$ -4) and ICT (lures > 1 stand deviation).[23] Healthy controls ($n = 308$) completed the Off and On state an average of 138 seconds, whereas patients with MHE completed the task an average of 198 seconds. When using PHES, the EncephalApp had sensitivity and specificity of 80% and 61%, respectively. Of note, the studies of EncephalApp excluded patients with alcohol use in the past 3 to 6 months as well as those on psychoactive drugs that were not on stable antidepressants.

Despite the ease of EncephalApp-Stroop test, the use outside of clinical trials in real-world settings has been low at nearly 32%,[24] suggesting that the onus of screening and monitoring of MHE cannot solely rely on the patient or caregiver. More recently and even shorter version of the EncephalApp-Stroop test, the Quick-Stroop found that decreasing the test time to just two runs (which can be accomplished in less than 1 minute), in the "Off state" was statistically equivalent to the entire EncephalApp-Stroop test, using PHES as the gold standard for diagnosis.[25] This ultra-short version may be easier for patients to complete during a clinic visit, but the barriers of downloading a smartphone application still exist.

The animal naming test

Part of the original Repeatable Battery for Assessment of Neuropsychological Status, the animal naming test is a shortened version taking 1 minute to complete without any tools needed. The animal naming test also does not require a trained clinician to score or interpret. It was initially studied and validated in Italy by Campagna and colleagues using patients admitted to two hospitals compared with healthy individuals and patients with inflammatory bowel disease also admitted to the hospital.[26] The PHES test (score ≤ -4) was used as the gold standard for diagnosis of MHE. The test requires simply asking a subject to name as many animals as they can in 1-minute animal naming test 1 (ANT_1). The test is influenced negatively by age (>80 year old) and education (<8 years) and was therefore adjusted to take into account these factors (S-ANT_1). The scores were correlated with PHES and EEG. In patients with cirrhosis, an simplified animal naming test 1 (S-$ANTI_1$) score of less than 10 animals was associated with future development of overt encephalopathy.[26] Furthermore, a recent prospective cohort study in the United States using the S-ANT_1 animal naming test found increased frailty and disability in patients who scored poorly, strengthening the concept that this is a clinically relevant test.[27]

Potential use of risk scores and predictive modeling for minimal hepatic encephalopathy

Because diagnosing MHE can be quite challenging, a shift to developing risk scores for development of overt HE may be a valid alternative approach. Risk scores and predictive modeling have become an integral part of health care in multiple settings.

BABS score

A retrospective cohort study over 5 years of veteran patients with cirrhosis was used to create the BABS score: *B*ilirubin, *A*lbumin, nonselective *B*eta blocker use, *S*tatin use.[28] The BABS score was created to risk stratify patients with cirrhosis for development of OHE. Patients were analyzed if they had diagnostic codes for cirrhosis or a portal hypertensive complication and were excluded if their chart revealed prior diagnosis of hepatic encephalopathy or use of medications such as rifaximin and lactulose. The primary outcome was development of overt HE over the 5-year period. Multivariate analysis showed the use of statin was associated with lower risk of developing overt HE, whereas the use of nonselective beta blockade was associated with higher risk of developing overt HE.

Baseline bilirubin and albumin also had significant hazard ratios and were included in the score. Using these four variables, a risk score was created. Patients can score in one of three categories based on their baseline risk score: ≤ -10 low risk, -9 to 20 intermediate risk, and ≥ 21 high risk.[28] For patients with baseline low-risk scores, their risk of developing overt HE in the next 5 years was 27%. Patients with intermediate- or high-risk scores had 49% risk of developing overt HE at 5 years. Although the population studied, 98% male and 74% white, is not inclusive, a high BABS could be a clinical tool to screen for MHE, in addition to help counsel patients regarding falls and driving.

MELD-Na-activity-chair stands-quality of life hepatic encephalopathy score

Another relevant study to MHE evaluated cirrhotic patient's health- HRQOL using the self-reported Short Form-8 and Work Productivity and Activity Impairment questionnaire.[29]

The study also incorporated measurement of frailty using chair-stands within 30 seconds and combined these measurements with MELD-Na+ to create a new score, the MELD-Na-Activity-Chair Stands-Quality of Life Hepatic Encephalopathy (MASQ-HE).[29] The area under the receiver operating curve was 0.82 to predict overt HE development at 12 months. As the BABS score outlined above, The MASQ-HE and other risk scores for transition to overt HE require further validation, in particular regarding stratification by presence/absence of MHE, a factor which likely has major modulatory influence in the performance of tests and scores to predict the development of overt HE.

Artificial intelligence and digital biomarkers: cognition

It has been over 20 years since PHES was initially published as a diagnostic tool for MHE. Despite advances over the past few decades, there remains a need for an easily accessible, minimally invasive, and low-cost tool to diagnose MHE. The tools described above still require active implementation and participation by providers and patients. With decreasing patient encounter time, it is becoming necessary to shift the burden of diagnostics away from the clinician, medical staff, caretakers, and patients.

The use of artificial intelligence (AI) has the potential to expedite clinical diagnosis and shift toward more personalized and precise medicine. This is an opportunity to use natural language processing to evaluate subtle changes in cognition during patient encounters.[30]

Dickerson and colleagues published a retrospective pilot study on pretransplant and posttransplant individuals compared with control and found that patient-generated EMR messages to health care team had slight differences in lexical and syntactic domains that may capture MHE.[31] There is increasing use of electronic medical record software that records patient encounters to aid in documentation and billing. The rate of speech has been evaluated as a biomarker and one study found that low psychometric scores using PHES were correlated with significantly slowed speech.[32] Likely there will be rapid advancements in AI over the next decade to aid in diagnostics, perhaps making many of the current tools to assess MHE obsolete.

Management of Minimal Hepatic Encephalopathy

The management of MHE presents a challenge due to the difficulties in establishing a definitive diagnosis. As outlined above, evaluation and interpretation of a range of psychometric tests, changes in clinical symptoms, and laboratory data have been suggested to accurately recognize, identify, and ultimately diagnose MHE. Despite a lack of consensus on therapeutic strategies for MHE and controversies on potential benefits and risks, the pursuit of novel prevention or reversal strategies has sparked numerous clinical trials. Several studies have explored MHE treatment, primarily based on variations of established therapies for overt HE. The current options for managing MHE include interventions to alter the intestinal microbiota with nonabsorbable disaccharides such as lactulose, nonabsorbable antibiotics such as rifaximin, probiotics, fecal microbiota transplantation (FMT), L-ornithine L-aspartate (LOLA), and maintaining proper nutritional status while averting sarcopenia with branched-chain amino acids (BCAAs) and a high protein diet[33–35] (**Box 4**).

Nonabsorbable disaccharides

Nonabsorbable disaccharides, including lactulose and lactitol, are currently the primary treatment for OHE (and covert stage I HE) and exert their effect through various mechanisms, including osmotic laxative effect, lowering of intraluminal pH levels, and modulation of gut microbiome.

By shortening colonic transit time, lactulose decreases the amount of time that gut bacteria are exposed to nutrients and substrates, thereby reducing ammonia production. In addition, lactulose can lower intraluminal pH levels, which in turn prevents the conversion of $NH4+$ ammonium cation to $NH3+$ ammonia. As $NH4+$ ammonium is not readily absorbed, it is excreted in the feces, further reducing the amount of

> **Box 4**
> **Therapeutic interventions for patients with minimal hepatic encephalopathy and potential agents which require of additional evaluation**
>
> Therapeutic Interventions for Patients with Minimal Hepatic Encephalopathy
> - Lactulose and other nonabsorbable disaccharides
> - Probiotics
> - Rifaximin
>
> Potential Agents which Require of Additional Evaluation
> - Polyethylene glycol (PEG)
> - Fecal microbiota transplantation (FMT)
> - L-ornithine L-aspartate (LOLA)
> - Branched-chain amino acids

ammonia produced. Another mechanism by which nonabsorbable disaccharides reduce ammonia production is through modulation of the gut microbiome. Disaccharides are metabolized by the gut microbiome, leading to a reduction in ammonia-producing microbiota due to the low pH acidic environment. As a result, there is a decrease in the amount of ammonia produced in the colon, which can be associated with lower blood ammonia levels.[36]

Several clinical studies have explored the efficacy of lactulose in the management of MHE.[37,38] In a pioneer clinical trial, McClain and colleagues demonstrated the effectiveness of lactulose in improving psychomotor performance in patients with alcohol-associated cirrhosis who did not exhibit overt HE.[39] The study comprised 32 patients who were randomly assigned to receive either lactulose or sucrose daily for a period of 3 months. Of note, patients treated with lactulose showed significant improvements in the Reitan trail test, writing speed, and digit symbol test, whereas no significant improvement was observed in the sucrose group.[39] Watanabe and colleagues also demonstrated the efficacy of lactulose treatment in improving psychometric tests, such as the NCT, symbol digit, and BDTs of the Wechsler adult intelligence scale, in patients with MHE.[40]

The study included 22 MHE patients who received lactulose (45 mL/d) for 8 weeks, whereas 14 did not receive lactulose. The lactulose treatment group exhibited significant improvements in psychometric evaluations at 4 and 8 weeks, with 50% of patients experiencing resolution of MHE by week 8, compared with 85% of untreated patients who had persistent MHE.[40] Prasad and colleagues investigated the effect of lactulose treatment on HRQOL and cognitive functions in cirrhotic patients with MHE[41]; 61 patients with MHE were randomly assigned in a 1:1 ratio to receive treatment (lactulose) for 3 months or no treatment. The results showed that lactulose improved both cognitive function and HRQOL compared with the untreated group, and the improvement in HRQOL was related to the improvement in psychometry.[41]

Thus, a trial of lactulose should be considered in patients with cirrhosis who complain of falls, driving difficulties, experience traffic accidents or violations, or have a decreased quality of life and test positive for MHE (see **Boxes 2** and **3**).

Rifaximin

Rifaximin, a semisynthetic derivative of the naturally occurring antibiotic rifamycin exhibits a broad spectrum anti-microbial activity against both gram-positive and gram-negative bacterial intestinal flora. Rifaximin inhibits bacterial RNA synthesis via its binding to the beta subunit of bacterial DNA-dependent RNA polymerase ultimately suppressing bacterial protein synthesis.

It has minimal systemic absorption, acting locally within the intestinal tract, targeting bacterial overgrowth and lowering bacterial toxins production.[42,43] Rifaximin also has anti-inflammatory activity, inhibiting the activation of pro-inflammatory cytokines and reducing intestinal permeability, thereby preventing translocation of harmful substances from the gut into the systemic compartments.[44,45]

Multiple clinical trials, reviewed elsewhere in this Clinics in Liver Disease Issue, have established clear roles for rifaximin in the management of overt HE. Consequently, rifaximin has emerged as a potential treatment option for the management of MHE as well.[33–35] Bajaj and colleagues showed that patients with MHE exhibited significant improvements in driving simulator performance following treatment with rifaximin, compared with those who received a placebo.[46] Rifaximin was associated with enhanced cognitive function and reduced endotoxemia in MHE patients in another study.[47] These findings were accompanied by changes in relationships between gut microbiome.[46,47]

Unproven but Potentially Helpful Therapies for Minimal Hepatic Encephalopathy

Polyethylene glycol

Polyethylene glycol (PEG) is a water-soluble, nonabsorbable, nontoxic polymer which is used as an osmotic laxative to treat constipation or colon purge before colonoscopy. PEG is not absorbed and passes through the gastrointestinal tract unaltered, increasing the water content of the stools.[48] PEG has been extensively evaluated for overt HE,[49–52] but to our knowledge, no clinical trial has investigated the efficacy and safety of PEG as a treatment for MHE. In the overt HE setting, PEG is used sometimes in conjunction with lower doses of lactulose, or without lactulose, in patients who are unable to tolerate lactulose.[52] Because of its laxative effect, PEG could be a potentially useful agent in MHE. A prospective evaluation of PEG, which is available over the counter in the United States, as a possible therapeutic tool for MHE seems a reasonable research endeavor.

Probiotics

Probiotics are live bacteria beneficial to the gut microbiota which have been studied for a potential therapeutic role in the treatment of MHE. Dysbiosis, an imbalance in the gut microbiota, has been linked to the development and progression of hepatic encephalopathy in cirrhosis. Probiotics restore gut microbiota equilibrium, effectively reducing the production and absorption of various toxic molecules, including ammonia. Another notable benefit of probiotics is their ability to enhance gut barrier function. Bacterial translocation, a pathologic process involving migration of gut bacteria into the systemic circulation, can incite inflammation and endotoxemia, both of which are pathogenetic mechanisms for hepatic encephalopathy.

Furthermore, probiotics exhibit immunomodulatory effects within the gut by attenuating the activity of immune-mediated cells, thereby contributing to a reduction in inflammation. Given the role of inflammation in the pathogenesis of hepatic encephalopathy, this immunomodulatory action highlights the potential benefits of probiotics in the management of HE.[53–55]

In a randomized controlled trial conducted by Malaguarnera and colleagues, the efficacy of Bifidobacterium longum with fructo-oligosaccharide was investigated in patients diagnosed with MHE.[56] Following a 90-day treatment period, the group receiving Bifidobacterium showed a significant decrease in serum ammonia levels, along with notable improvement in performance on both the Symbol Digit Modalities Test (SDMT) and BDT, indicative of enhanced cognitive function.[35] Bajaj and colleagues further demonstrated similar improvements in cognitive function using surrogate markers of MHE reversal, including BDT, SDMT, and NCT-A, in addition to showing excellent adherence to probiotic yogurt supplementation compare to the placebo group among nonalcoholic cirrhotic patients.[57]

In a small prospective, open-label, randomized study, Manzhalii studied the safety and efficacy of Escherichia coli Nissle (EcN) 1917 strain compared with lactulose and rifaximin. EcN was found non-inferior to rifaximin; however, it outperformed lactulose in terms of ammonia and pro-inflammatory cytokines reduction, gut microbiota modulation and cognitive function improvement among patients with MHE.[58]

In summary, probiotics for MHE seem promising and have excellent adherence but further studies are needed to identify their granular benefits, best type of probiotics, and optimal dose and administration program for MHE.

Fecal microbiota transplantation

FMT involves transferring fecal material from a healthy donor to a patient suffering from gut dysbiosis, using methods such as a nasoduodenal tube, enema, or colonoscopy. FMT is now integrated into mainstream medicine.[59,60]

Cirrhotic patients with MHE have distinct changes in gut microbiota patterns, with reduced levels of certain short-chain fatty acid-producing Firmicutes, including Lachnospiraceae and Ruminococcaceae and abundance of proteobacteria, such as Enterobacteriaceae.[61] Based on this information, Bajaj and colleagues conducted an open-label, randomized controlled trial involving a single stool donor with abundant Lachnospiraceae and Ruminococcaceae, identified by a machine learning technique[62]; 10 participants received FMT via enema and 10 control subjects received lactulose and rifaximin as standard of care. The trial outcomes were favorable as FMT from the rationally selected donor reduced hospitalizations, improved cognition and dysbiosis in cirrhotic patients with recurrent HE.[46]

Safety and improvements in clinical and cognitive function parameters among patients treated with FMT enemas were sustained in the long term (>12 months).[62,63] These investigators also found that patients preferred FMT capsules over enema.[64]

To our knowledge, FMT has not been studied specifically in the management of MHE. The progress in FMT formulation (capsules), coupled with the recent FDA approval of a commercially available, rectally administered FMT agent in 2022, is expected to enhance accessibility to FMT therapy. Given the unmet needs in MHE therapy, further evaluation of FMT as a potential intervention for patients with MHE seems warranted.

ʟ-ornithine ʟ-aspartate

LOLA is a combination of two amino acids with potential therapeutic use in the management of hepatic encephalopathy and other metabolic disorders characterized by hyperammonemia. ʟ-ornithine activates glutamine synthetase activity and promotes glutamine synthesis and because glutamine is the main reservoir of ammonia in the liver, it ameliorates hyperammonemia. On the other hand, ʟ-aspartate is converted to urea in the liver. Thus, LOLA alleviates hepatic encephalopathy by lowering ammonia production by multiple mechanisms,[65,66] and indeed, numerous randomized controlled trials have documented the efficacy of LOLA in the management of overt episodic or chronic HE.[67,68]

Mittal and colleagues studied the efficacy of LOLA (6g three times daily) in the management of 160 patients with MHE.[69] LOLA significantly improved HRQOL and lowered arterial ammonia level in patients with MHE compared with no treatment.[69] Similarly, another study found that MHE patients who received LOLA treatment exhibited notable enhancement in neuropsychometric tests and critical flicker frequency results, in comparison to those who were administered placebo.[70] LOLA and lactulose were most effective in preventing transition to overt HE in patients with MHE on a recent systematic review of various treatment options for MHE[38] despite a prior Cochrane review of 36 randomized clinical trials in which subgroup analyses showed no differences in MHE outcomes associated with LOLA therapy.[71]

Branched-chain amino acids

The BCAAs, valine, leucine, and isoleucine play an important role in nitrogen metabolism and muscle protein synthesis. A Cochrane database systematic review of 16 randomized clinical trials concluded that BCAAs were beneficial in patients with overt HE.[72] However, as with other potential interventions outlined above, BCAAs have had very limited evaluation in the setting of MHE.[38,73]

In conclusion, multiple agents have been found to reverse the neurophysiological abnormalities of MHE, particularly lactulose and rifaximin, whereas others (lactulose, LOLA) seem to have the capability of decreasing transition to overt HE in patients with MHE. However, the adverse events of lactulose and the cost of rifaximin prevent recommending therapy for every patient with MHE. Current guidance suggests considering therapy for MHE on a case-by-case basis.[7] We interpret this to suggest a therapeutic trial in cirrhotic patients with falls, motor vehicle accidents, machine operators, subjective feelings of neurologic deficits, or employment difficulties. Lactulose seems the first-line treatment for MHE due to its strong evidence of effectiveness in improving both MHE and HRQOL. A trial of lactulose is reasonable in patients with cirrhosis who complain of falls, driving difficulties, experience traffic accidents and violations, or have a decreased quality of life and test positive for MHE (see **Boxes 2** and **3**). In cases of MHE recurrence or patients unresponsive to lactulose, rifaximin may serve as the second-line treatment, if financially feasible. For patients experiencing lactulose intolerance, an alternative option is the use of PEG, either as a substitute for lactulose or in combination with a reduced lactulose dose, understanding that PEG has not been evaluated in, or is formally indicated in MHE. A trial with probiotics is also an attractive option. Third-line agents, such as FMT, LOLA, and BCAAs, while generally safe in other settings, should be considered experimental and require the appropriate clinical trials to establish their role, if any, in the management of MHE.

CLINICS CARE POINTS

- Minimal hepatic encephalopathy is common in patients with cirrhosis.
- The standard neurological examination is normal in patients with minimal encephalopathy.
- The Animal Naming Test and EncephalApp-Stroop tests are useful to screen for minimal encephalopathy in the office or bedside setttings.
- A trial of lactulose or probiotics can be considered for patients with minimal encephalopathy.

DISCLOSURE

The authors have no commercial conflicts of interest and no funding sources connected with this article.

REFERENCES

1. Bajaj JS, Wade JB, Sanyal AJ. Spectrum of neurocognitive impairment in cirrhosis: Implications for the assessment of hepatic encephalopathy. Hepatology 2009;50(6):2014–21.

2. Weissenborn K, Ennen JC, Schomerus H, et al. Neuropsychological characterization of hepatic encephalopathy. J Hepatol 2001;34(5):768–73.
3. Bajaj JS, Cordoba J, Mullen KD, et al. Review article: the design of clinical trials in hepatic encephalopathy–an International Society for Hepatic Encephalopathy and Nitrogen Metabolism (ISHEN) consensus statement. Aliment Pharmacol Ther 2011;33(7):739–47.
4. Bajaj JS, Duarte-Rojo A, Xie JJ, et al. Minimal hepatic encephalopathy and mild cognitive impairment worsen quality of life in Elderly patients with cirrhosis. Clin Gastroenterol Hepatol 2020;18(13):3008–e2.
5. Bajaj JS, Saeian K, Schubert CM, et al. Minimal hepatic encephalopathy is associated with motor vehicle crashes: the reality beyond the driving test. Hepatology 2009;50(4):1175–83.
6. Bajaj JS. Minimal hepatic encephalopathy matters in daily life. World J Gastroenterol 2008;14(23):3609–15.
7. Vilstrup H, Amodio P, Bajaj J, et al. Hepatic encephalopathy in chronic liver disease: 2014 practice guideline by the American association for the study of liver diseases and the European association for the study of the liver. Hepatology 2014;60(2):715–35.
8. Campagna F, Montagnese S, Schiff S, et al. Cognitive impairment and electroencephalographic alterations before and after liver transplantation: what is reversible? Liver Transpl 2014;20(8):977–86.
9. Gairing SJ, Schleicher EM, Galle PR, et al. Prediction and prevention of the first episode of overt hepatic encephalopathy in patients with cirrhosis. Hepatol Commun 2023;7(4).
10. Bai M, Qi XS, Yang ZP, et al. TIPS improves liver transplantation-free survival in cirrhotic patients with refractory ascites: an updated meta-analysis. World J Gastroenterol 2014;20(10):2704–14.
11. Tapper EB, Parikh ND, Waljee AK, et al. Diagnosis of minimal hepatic encephalopathy: a systematic review of point-of-care diagnostic tests. Am J Gastroenterol 2018;113(4):529–38.
12. Bajaj JS, Lauridsen M, Tapper EB, et al. Important Unresolved questions in the management of hepatic encephalopathy: an ISHEN consensus. Am J Gastroenterol 2020;115(7):989–1002.
13. Luo M, Ma P, Li L, et al. Advances in psychometric tests for screening minimal hepatic encephalopathy: from paper-and-pencil to computer-aided assessment. Turk J Gastroenterol 2019;30(5):398–407.
15. Nabi E, Thacker LR, Wade JB, et al. Diagnosis of covert hepatic encephalopathy without specialized tests. Clin Gastroenterol Hepatol 2014;12(8):1384–e2.
14. Lauridsen MM, Jepsen P, Wernberg CW, et al. Validation of a simple quality-of-life score for Identification of minimal and prediction of overt hepatic encephalopathy. Hepatol Commun 2020;4(9):1353–61.
16. Bajaj JS, Saeian K, Verber MD, et al. Inhibitory control test is a simple method to diagnose minimal hepatic encephalopathy and predict development of overt hepatic encephalopathy. Am J Gastroenterol 2007;102(4):754–60.
17. Bajaj JS, Hafeezullah M, Franco J, et al. Inhibitory control test for the diagnosis of minimal hepatic encephalopathy. Gastroenterology 2008;135(5):1591–e1.
18. Stawicka A, Jaroszewicz J, Zbrzeźniak J, et al. Clinical Usefulness of the inhibitory control test (ICT) in the diagnosis of minimal hepatic encephalopathy. Int J Environ Res Public Health 2020;17(10):3645.
19. Khan H, Rauch A, Obolsky M, et al. A comparison of embedded validity indicators from the Stroop Color and Word Test among adults referred for clinical

evaluation of suspected or confirmed attention-deficit/hyperactivity disorder. Psychol Assess 2022;34(7):697–703.

20. Felipo V, Ordoño JF, Urios A, et al. Patients with minimal hepatic encephalopathy show impaired mismatch negativity correlating with reduced performance in attention tests. Hepatology 2012;55(2):530–9.

21. Bajaj JS, Thacker LR, Heuman DM, et al. The Stroop smartphone application is a short and valid method to screen for minimal hepatic encephalopathy. Hepatology 2013;58(3):1122–32.

22. Bajaj JS, Heuman DM, Sterling RK, et al. Validation of EncephalApp, smartphone-based Stroop test, for the diagnosis of covert hepatic encephalopathy. Clin Gastroenterol Hepatol 2015;13(10):1828–e1.

23. Allampati S, Duarte-Rojo A, Thacker LR, et al. Diagnosis of minimal hepatic encephalopathy using Stroop EncephalApp: a multicenter US-based, Norm-based study. Am J Gastroenterol 2016;111(1):78–86.

24. Louissaint J, Lok AS, Fortune BE, et al. Acceptance and use of a smartphone application in cirrhosis. Liver Int 2020;40(7):1556–63.

25. Acharya C, Shaw J, Duong N, et al. QuickStroop, a shortened version of EncephalApp, detects covert hepatic encephalopathy with similar accuracy within one minute. Clin Gastroenterol Hepatol 2023;21(1):136–42.

26. Campagna F, Montagnese S, Ridola L, et al. The animal naming test: an easy tool for the assessment of hepatic encephalopathy. Hepatology 2017;66(1):198–208.

27. Tapper EB, Kenney B, Nikirk S, et al. Animal naming test is associated with poor patient-reported outcomes and frailty in people with and without cirrhosis: a prospective cohort study. Clin Transl Gastroenterol 2022;13(1):e00447.

28. Tapper EB, Parikh ND, Sengupta N, et al. A risk score to predict the development of hepatic encephalopathy in a population-based cohort of patients with cirrhosis. Hepatology 2018;68(4):1498–507.

29. Tapper EB, Zhao L, Nikirk S, et al. Incidence and Bedside Predictors of the first episode of overt hepatic encephalopathy in patients with cirrhosis. Am J Gastroenterol 2020;115(12):2017–25.

30. Sprint G, Cook DJ, Schmitter-Edgecombe M, et al. Multimodal Fusion of smart home and Text-based behavior markers for clinical assessment prediction. ACM Trans Comput Healthc 2022;3(4).

31. Dickerson LK, Rouhizadeh M, Korotkaya Y, et al. Language impairment in adults with end-stage liver disease: application of natural language processing towards patient-generated health records. NPJ Digit Med 2019;2:106.

32. Moon AM, Kim HP, Cook S, et al. Speech patterns and enunciation for encephalopathy determination-A prospective study of hepatic encephalopathy. Hepatol Commun 2022;6(10):2876–85.

33. Karanfilian BV, Park T, Senatore F, et al. Minimal hepatic encephalopathy. Clin Liver Dis 2020;24(2):209–18.

34. Rudler M, Weiss N, Bouzbib C, et al. Diagnosis and management of hepatic encephalopathy. Clin Liver Dis 2021;25(2):393–417.

35. Badal BD, Bajaj JS. Hepatic encephalopathy: diagnostic tools and management strategies. Med Clin North Am 2023;107(3):517–31.

36. Elwir S, Rahimi RS. Hepatic encephalopathy: an Update on the Pathophysiology and therapeutic options. J Clin Transl Hepatol 2017;5(2):142–51.

37. Als-Nielsen B, Gluud LL, Gluud C. Nonabsorbable disaccharides for hepatic encephalopathy. Cochrane Database Syst Rev 2004;(2):CD003044. :CD003044.

38. Dhiman RK, Thumburu KK, Verma N, et al. Comparative efficacy of treatment options for minimal hepatic encephalopathy: a systematic review and Network meta-analysis. Clin Gastroenterol Hepatol 2020;18(4):800–e25.
39. McClain CJ, Potter TJ, Kromhout JP, et al. The effect of lactulose on psychomotor performance tests in alcoholic cirrhotics without overt hepatic encephalopathy. J Clin Gastroenterol 1984;6(4):325–9.
40. Watanabe A, Sakai T, Sato S, et al. Clinical efficacy of lactulose in cirrhotic patients with and without subclinical hepatic encephalopathy. Hepatology 1997; 26(6):1410–4.
41. Prasad S, Dhiman RK, Duseja A, et al. Lactulose improves cognitive functions and health-related quality of life in patients with cirrhosis who have minimal hepatic encephalopathy. Hepatology 2007;45(3):549–59.
42. Testa R, Eftimiadi C, Sukkar GS, et al. A non-absorbable rifamycin for treatment of hepatic encephalopathy. Drugs Exp Clin Res 1985;11(6):387–92.
43. Venturini AP, Marchi E. In vitro and in vivo evaluation of L/105, a new topical intestinal rifamycin. Chemioterapia 1986;5(4):257–62.
44. Mencarelli A, Renga B, Palladino G, et al. Inhibition of NF-κB by a PXR-dependent pathway mediates counter-regulatory activities of rifaximin on innate immunity in intestinal epithelial cells. Eur J Pharmacol 2011;668(1–2):317–24.
45. Fiorucci S, Distrutti E, Mencarelli A, et al. Inhibition of intestinal bacterial translocation with rifaximin modulates lamina propria monocytic cells reactivity and protects against inflammation in a rodent model of colitis. Digestion 2002;66(4): 246–56.
46. Bajaj JS, Heuman DM, Wade JB, et al. Rifaximin improves driving simulator performance in a randomized trial of patients with minimal hepatic encephalopathy. Gastroenterology 2011;140(2):478–e1.
47. Bajaj JS, Heuman DM, Sanyal AJ, et al. Modulation of the metabiome by rifaximin in patients with cirrhosis and minimal hepatic encephalopathy. PLoS One 2013; 8(4):e60042.
48. DiPalma JA, Brady CE 3rd. Colon cleansing for diagnostic and surgical procedures: polyethylene glycol-electrolyte lavage solution. Am J Gastroenterol 1989; 84(9):1008–16.
49. Rahimi RS, Singal AG, Cuthbert JA, et al. Lactulose vs polyethylene glycol 3350–electrolyte solution for treatment of overt hepatic encephalopathy: the HELP randomized clinical trial. JAMA Intern Med 2014;174(11):1727–33.
50. Shehata HH, Elfert AA, Abdin AA, et al. Randomized controlled trial of polyethylene glycol versus lactulose for the treatment of overt hepatic encephalopathy. Eur J Gastroenterol Hepatol 2018;30(12):1476–81.
51. Naderian M, Akbari H, Saeedi M, et al. Polyethylene glycol and lactulose versus lactulose Alone in the treatment of hepatic encephalopathy in patients with cirrhosis: a non-Inferiority randomized controlled trial. Middle East J Dig Dis 2017;9(1):12–9.
52. Ahmed S, Premkumar M, Dhiman RK, et al. Combined PEG3350 Plus lactulose results in early resolution of hepatic encephalopathy and improved 28-day survival in Acute-on-chronic liver Failure. J Clin Gastroenterol 2022;56(1):e11–9.
53. Cesaro C, Tiso A, Del Prete A, et al. Gut microbiota and probiotics in chronic liver diseases. Dig Liver Dis 2011;43(6):431–8.
54. Dhiman RK. Gut microbiota and hepatic encephalopathy. Metab Brain Dis 2013; 28(2):321–6.
55. Arab JP, Martin-Mateos RM, Shah VH. Gut-liver axis, cirrhosis and portal hypertension: the chicken and the egg. Hepatol Int 2018;12(Suppl 1):24–33.

56. Malaguarnera M, Greco F, Barone G, et al. Bifidobacterium longum with fructo-oligosaccharide (FOS) treatment in minimal hepatic encephalopathy: a random-ized, double-blind, placebo-controlled study. Dig Dis Sci 2007;52(11):3259–65.

57. Bajaj JS, Saeian K, Christensen KM, et al. Probiotic yogurt for the treatment of minimal hepatic encephalopathy. Am J Gastroenterol 2008;103(7):1707–15.

58. Manzhalii E, Moyseyenko V, Kondratiuk V, et al. Effect of a specific Escherichia coli Nissle 1917 strain on minimal/mild hepatic encephalopathy treatment. World J Hepatol 2022;14(3):634–46.

59. Stripling J, Rodriguez M. Current evidence in Delivery and therapeutic Uses of fecal microbiota transplantation in human diseases-Clostridium difficile disease and beyond. Am J Med Sci 2018;356(5):424–32.

60. van Nood E, Vrieze A, Nieuwdorp M, et al. Duodenal infusion of donor feces for recurrent Clostridium difficile. N Engl J Med 2013;368(5):407–15.

61. Bajaj JS, Heuman DM, Hylemon PB, et al. Altered profile of human gut micro-biome is associated with cirrhosis and its complications. J Hepatol 2014;60(5):940–7.

62. Bajaj JS, Kassam Z, Fagan A, et al. Fecal microbiota transplant from a rational stool donor improves hepatic encephalopathy: a randomized clinical trial. Hepa-tology 2017;66(6):1727–38.

63. Bajaj JS, Fagan A, Gavis EA, et al. Long-term outcomes of fecal microbiota trans-plantation in patients with cirrhosis. Gastroenterology 2019;156(6):1921–e3.

64. Bajaj JS, Salzman NH, Acharya C, et al. Fecal microbial transplant capsules are safe in hepatic encephalopathy: a Phase 1, randomized, placebo-controlled trial. Hepatology 2019;70(5):1690–703.

65. Kaiser S, Gerok W, Häussinger D. Ammonia and glutamine metabolism in human liver slices: new aspects on the pathogenesis of hyperammonaemia in chronic liver disease. Eur J Clin Invest 1988;18(5):535–42.

66. Stoll B, McNelly S, Buscher HP, et al. Functional hepatocyte heterogeneity in glutamate, aspartate and alpha-ketoglutarate uptake: a histoautoradiographical study. Hepatology 1991;13(2):247–53.

67. Gebhardt R, Beckers G, Gaunitz F, et al. Treatment of cirrhotic rats with L-orni-thine-L-aspartate enhances urea synthesis and lowers serum ammonia levels. J Pharmacol Exp Ther 1997;283(1):1–6.

68. Kircheis G, Nilius R, Held C, et al. Therapeutic efficacy of L-ornithine-L-aspartate infusions in patients with cirrhosis and hepatic encephalopathy: results of a placebo-controlled, double-blind study. Hepatology 1997;25(6):1351–60.

69. Mittal VV, Sharma BC, Sharma P, et al. A randomized controlled trial comparing lactulose, probiotics, and L-ornithine L-aspartate in treatment of minimal hepatic encephalopathy. Eur J Gastroenterol Hepatol 2011;23(8):725–32.

70. Sharma K, Pant S, Misra S, et al. Effect of rifaximin, probiotics, and l-ornithine l-aspartate on minimal hepatic encephalopathy: a randomized controlled trial. Saudi J Gastroenterol 2014;20(4):225–32.

71. Goh ET, Stokes CS, Sidhu SS, et al. L-ornithine L-aspartate for prevention and treatment of hepatic encephalopathy in people with cirrhosis. Cochrane Data-base Syst Rev 2018;5(5):CD012410.

72. Gluud LL, Dam G, Les I, et al. Branched-chain amino acids for people with hepat-ic encephalopathy. Cochrane Database Syst Rev 2017;5(5):CD001939.

73. Plauth M, Egberts E, Hamster W, et al. Long-term treatment of latent portosyste-mic encephalopathy with branched-chain amino acids. A double-blind placebo-controlled crossover study. J Hepatol 1993;17:308–14.

Hepatic Encephalopathy
Clinical Manifestations

Kabiru Ohikere, MD, MHA[a], Robert J. Wong, MD, MS[b,c],*

KEYWORDS

- Clinical manifestations • Hepatic encephalopathy • West Haven

KEY POINTS

- Hepatic encephalopathy (HE) can occur as a complication of chronic liver disease as well as acute liver failure.
- HE can present across a spectrum of severity, from early covert symptoms that may only be accurately detected with careful attention and specialized testing to overt symptoms that often accompany the development of liver decompensation and/or liver failure.
- Timely identification of HE is critical so that appropriate treatment can be implemented in a timely fashion.

INTRODUCTION

Hepatic encephalopathy (HE) is a serious complication that can develop in patients with chronic liver diseases, cirrhosis, and patients who present with acute liver failure.[1–3] Concurrent HE is particularly concerning and deserving of greater attention because most patients who develop HE have already developed advanced liver disease with impaired synthetic function and/or hepatic decompensation and are a high risk for further decompensation, contributing the liver-related morbidity and mortality.[2,3] Similarly, HE most commonly develops in patients who have already developed cirrhosis that has progressed to clinically significant portal hypertension, and hence the need for early diagnosis and early implementation of HE treatment in these critically ill patients (**Table 1**).[4] Our current understanding is that the development of HE is primarily driven by 2 main mechanisms of action: liver insufficiency and portal-systemic shunting.[2,3] These mechanisms and how they uniquely contribute to the pathogenesis and clinical manifestations of HE will be discussed further in this article as well as other supporting articles.

a Value Based Care Department, San Francisco Health Network / Zuckerberg San Francisco General Hospital and Trauma Center; b Division of Gastroenterology and Hepatology, Stanford University School of Medicine; c Gastroenterology Section, Veterans Affairs Palo Alto Healthcare System, Palo Alto, CA, USA
* Corresponding author. 3801 Miranda Avenue GI-111, Palo Alto, CA 94304.
E-mail address: rwong123@stanford.edu

Clin Liver Dis 28 (2024) 253–263
https://doi.org/10.1016/j.cld.2024.01.005
1089-3261/24/Published by Elsevier Inc.
liver.theclinics.com

Table 1 Proposed nomenclature of hepatic encephalopathy[4]			
Type	Encephalopathy Associated With	Subcategory	Subdivisions
A	Acute liver failure		
B	Portal-systemic bypass and no intrinsic hepatocellular disease		
C	Cirrhosis and portal hypertension and/or portal-systemic shunts	Episodic	Precipitated Spontaneous[a] Recurrent[b]
		Persistent[c]	Mild (grade 1) Severe (grades 2–4) Treatment-dependent
		Minimal	

[a] Without recognized precipitating factors.
[b] Recurrent = 2 episodes within 1 y
[c] Persistent = cognitive deficits that affect negatively on social and occupational functioning.

Recent studies evaluating epidemiology of cirrhosis and cirrhosis-related complications have reported an overall increasing prevalence of HE, which is likely a reflection of multiple contributing factors.[5–8] Existing data have demonstrated overall increasing burden of patients with chronic liver disease, especially those with advanced liver disease that are at higher risk of developing liver-related complications such as HE.[7–9] This is largely driven by the aging population of patients with chronic liver disease, compounded by the continued increasing prevalence of individuals with metabolic dysfunction associated steatotic liver disease (MASLD) and metabolic dysfunction associated steatohepatitis (MASH).[10–14] More recent epidemiology data also report on increasing clinical burden of alcohol-related liver diseases, including alcohol-associated hepatitis and alcohol-associated cirrhosis, all of which has further fueled the increase in the prevalence of patients with advanced liver disease and liver-related complications.[9,15–19] These trends further emphasize the importance of early identification and timely treatment of liver-related complications. In particular, increased awareness of diagnostic modalities to improve early identification and treatment of HE is needed as well as improved management of patients with cirrhosis and HE-related complications.[1–3] In the subsequent sections, we briefly review updates in the epidemiology of HE, provide a summary of current diagnostic modalities for identifying HE and assessing HE severity, and provide a detailed discussion about the clinical manifestations of patients with HE.

EPIDEMIOLOGY OF HEPATIC ENCEPHALOPATHY
Overview

Despite advancements in the treatment of chronic hepatitis C virus and chronic hepatitis B virus, the emerging burden of MASLD/MASH has contributed to increasing burden of cirrhosis. The prevalence of HE in this aging population of individuals with cirrhosis is increasing. From 2004 to 2014, there was a 1.10% per year percent increase in the prevalence of HE in patients aged 65 years and older.[5] Increasing burden of alcohol-associated liver disease (AALD) also has contributed to this increasing HE burden as heavy and chronic alcohol consumption in patients with AALD significantly affects the risk of HE. The incidence and prevalence of overt HE is higher in patients with alcohol-related cirrhosis than cirrhosis from other causes.[6,7,20] In a large population-based study that evaluated a 20% random sample of US Medicare enrollees with cirrhosis and Part D prescription coverage from 2008 to 2014, incidence and risk factors for HE were evaluated. Compared with MASLD, alcohol-related cirrhosis was found to be most strongly associated with incident HE.[6] In another prospective multicenter study of patients with biopsy proven MASLD in China, HE was the most frequent first decompensating event.[20]

Diabetes and glycemic control are also important risk factors for the development of HE in patients with cirrhosis, and in one study, comorbid diabetes was associated with an 86% increased risk of developing HE.[21,22] The autonomic neuropathy associated with diabetes can slow intestinal transit, promoting constipation and bacterial overgrowth.[23] Bacterial overgrowth along with increased bacterial translocation can further exacerbate the role of inflammation in the pathophysiology of HE.[24,25] Second, the kidneys are an important site for ammonia metabolism to glutamine; therefore, renal impairment from diabetic nephropathy promotes hyperammonemia and the risk of HE.[26] Third, the neurocognitive impact of diabetes, including increased permeability of the blood-brain barrier and neuro-inflammation related to hyperglycemia, can act synergistically with similar changes seen in HE.[27] Other risk factors associated with increased risk of HE include proton pump inhibitor use, chronic opiate use, and concurrent use of benzodiazepines.[6,28,29]

Although the incidence and prevalence of HE can be challenging to assess because of variation in the severity of the disease manifestations and the definition of HE (minimal vs overt), HE has been reported to occur in a wide range (20%–80%) of patients with cirrhosis.[30] The prevalence of overt HE at the time of cirrhosis diagnosis is approximately 10% to 14%. This increases to 16% to 21% in patients with decompensated cirrhosis and approximately 10% to 50% in patients who have undergone transjugular intrahepatic portosystemic shunt. Overall, an estimated 30% to 40% of patients with cirrhosis will experience overt HE during their clinical course.

Hospitalizations and Readmissions

Hospitalizations from the development of HE are quite common in patients with decompensated liver disease. Patients with chronic liver disease are also frequently admitted or readmitted for complications such as variceal bleeding, ascites, spontaneous bacterial peritonitis, and renal failure. Similar to HE, these other complications, although largely preventable, are associated with significant morbidity and mortality. The risks of readmissions for HE is increased in the presence of infections, dehydration, constipation, nonadherence to lactulose, high protein diet, and medications that alter mental status. In a US single-center, retrospective study (2011–2013) of 222 patients with decompensated cirrhosis, more than half (59.4%) were readmitted within a median 54 days, with HE identified most often as the cause for readmission (35.5%). In the aforementioned study, HE at the time of the index hospitalization was a significant predictor of shorter time to readmission and a significant predictor of readmission of 30 days or lesser.[31] Similarly, the presence of HE increased the odds of 30-day readmission in patients with cirrhosis from 3 US states included in the Hospital Readmissions Reduction Program between 2009 and 2013.[32] In another single center study (2008–2014), HE was specified as the cause for almost half of the 250 readmissions (45.4%).[33] Furthermore, patients with cirrhosis and a history of 1 to 3 infections were more likely to develop HE compared with those without a history of infections (adjusted OR, 2.68; 95% CI, 2.13–3.37; $P < .001$).[34]

Factors that may influence HE-related readmissions includes patient's socioeconomic status, level of education, income, and the patient's capacity for self-care. Patients with HE have impaired cognitive and affective capabilities that may lead to poor adherence with medication regimens and hospital follow-up visits. The residual effects of HE on cognitive function may result in learning impairment despite appropriate treatment.[35] Moreover, patients with even mild cognitive impairment may have a greater risk of hospitalization than patients with normal cognition.[36] Therefore, education of caregivers may be a strategy that can be used to reduce readmission in this high-risk group.

Impact on Health-Care Resource Utilization

HE-related complications and hospitalizations contribute to significant health-care economic burden as well. From 2010 to 2014, a 25% increase in hospitalizations for HE was found in an analysis using the National Inpatient Sample; this corresponds to nearly 700,000 HE-related hospitalizations.[8] During the same period, the cost of HE-related hospitalizations increased as well from US$1.8 billion in 2007 to US$2.33 billion in 2014. A recent analysis by Volk and colleagues using 2 large private insurance databases found an average cost of a hospital stay for HE to range from US$29,063 to US$34,810 during the study period (2014–2019).[37] Another data from the North American Consortium for the Study of End-Stage Liver Disease identified nearly one-quarter of all 90-day readmissions in cirrhosis were related to HE.[38]

Evaluation of Healthcare Cost and Utilization data during the past 11 years revealed some noteworthy trends. First, hospitalizations for HE are increasing. The number of hospital discharges for a primary diagnosis of HE was 17,266 in 1993, 23,482 in 1999, and 40,012 in 2003. Increases in the rate of hospital discharges also occurred for unspecified encephalopathy and cirrhosis. Second, cost per HE-related hospitalization has increased despite a decrease in the length of stay. The economic burden associated with minimal HE has not been fully investigated. However, impairment in mental, physical, and the patient's ability to work likely translates into substantial costs because of diminished work performance, lost wages for patients and their families and premature retirement.

A 30-day supply of rifaximin can cost more than US$2500, depending on insurance coverage. There are additional pharmacoequity concerns regarding disparities in access to this disease-modifying medication. In a recent study of United States Medicare enrollees, rifaximin use was lower among Black patients, who additionally paid more per prescription than White patients and were less likely to fill prescriptions because medication costs increased.[39,40] Still, it is cost-effective after factoring in a significant reduction in overall health-care costs, mainly related to fewer hospitalizations.[37,41]

HEPATIC ENCEPHALOPATHY: CLINICAL MANIFESTATIONS

The development of HE in acute liver failure can be a sign of severely impaired hepatic function, and the rapidity of HE progression can determine clinical outcomes for patients and the speed of recovery from the initial HE insult (**Box 1**). In patients where there is an indication for transplantation during an acute presentation, any delay in initiating such intervention can lead to feared outcomes such as cerebral edema, which is a major cause of mortality in patients with acute liver failure.[42] Patients with acute HE who maintain consciousness may present with exaggerated motor and tendon reflexes. There may be reappearance of primitive reflexes such as Babinski in some patients.[30] These increased reflexes can be diminished or lost in patients with progressive deterioration such as coma. Seizure activity is not commonly reported during episodes of acute HE.[43] Patients with fulminant hepatic failure without cirrhosis may experience worsening confusion, agitation, and may have body posture that points to an atraumatic brain injury such as decerebrate posturing.

In the subacute forms of HE or in less-severe presentations, patients may have cognitive impairment, attention deficit, psychomotor slowing, and, sometimes, an

> **Box 1**
> **Clinical manifestations of hepatic encephalopathy**
>
> - Impairment of consciousness (see **Table 2** WHC)
> - Exaggerated motor and tendon reflexes
> - Rigidity of muscles with resistance to passive motions
> - Reappearance of primitive reflexes such as Babinski
> - Psychomotor slowing
> - Attention deficit and slow response to conversation
> - Confusions and disorientation
> - Impaired memory with difficulty in recall
> - Overactivity and restlessness
> - Delusions
> - Repetitive picking movements

impaired capacity to drive. The constellation of these less-severe symptoms is termed minimal hepatic encephalopathy (MHE) and the presence of MHE increases the risk of progression to overt HE. The International Society for Hepatic Encephalopathy and Nitrogen Metabolism consensus defines the onset of disorientation or asterixis as the onset of overt hepatic encephalopathy (OHE).[44]

In pediatric acute liver failure (PALF) associated with HE, symptoms can also occur rapidly with accompanying coagulopathy and neuropsychiatric signs.[45] Although variability in observation and examination findings among pediatric group with HE do exist and may limit assessing for severity and outcomes, elevated serum neurologic markers such as neuron-specific enolase, major basic protein, and S 100β may be used to assess the development of HE in PALF but are not as reliable as the standard assessment test.[46–48]

Patients with compensated chronic liver disease or cirrhosis who develop HE may show signs of sleep disturbance. The alternation in sleep pattern can affect both the duration and quality of sleep. Some patients may have insomnia while others may experience excessive sleepiness during the day.[49,50] Intermittent awakenings at night have also been reported among patients with HE with background cirrhosis.[49,51] As the signs and symptoms of HE evolves, patients' personality can be adversely affected. Behavioral changes such as disinhibition, apathy, and irritability can become more prominent.[2] Neuropsychometric tests performed on patients may show impairment of memory, patient's ability to recall instructions, and their orientation.[52,53] Patient may also experience deteriorating attention span. Additionally, some musculoskeletal manifestations of HE may include rigidity, resting tremors, changed facies, and psychomotor retardation.[2]

In patients who are on portocaval shunting for extended period, another form of HE called hepatic myelopathy can occur. This myelopathy is described as having motor deficits such as paraplegia or spasticity that cannot be resolved with standard therapy, and with symptoms that outweighs the associated mental dysfunction.[54,55] Furthermore, extrapyramidal signs such as parkinsonism, dystonia, akathisia have also been seen in patients with chronic liver disease and cirrhosis.[56] Cirrhosis-associated parkinsonism is also said to be unresponsive to conventional agents that reduces the systemic absorption of ammonia in the gastrointestinal tract.

HEPATIC ENCEPHALOPATHY: GRADING AND TESTING

HE can be classified according to the severity of the presenting signs and symptoms, its time course, and if an episode of HE had an associated precipitating factor or not. Another classification used is based on the underlying disease, and more recently, whether the patient has an acute-on-chronic liver failure.[57] Observable signs such as asterixis and disorientation can serve as a marker of OHE.[58] Clinical scales such as the West Haven Criteria (WHC; **Table 2**) can be used to evaluate the severity of OHE. In situations where there is a pronounced alteration in the level of consciousness, the Glasgow Coma Scale can also be used to assess the severity of OHE. Patients with MHE or covert hepatic encephalopathy may be more challenging to evaluate because they have no physical signs of impairments for most times and would therefore depend on a more complex testing strategies for assessment. Several psychometric and neurophysiologic tests are available but no single one can completely evaluate the range of impairment that could potentially be uncovered in a patient with either MHE or CME.[59,60] To increase accuracy, the International Society for Hepatic Encephalopathy and Nitrogen Metabolism (ISHEN) recommends that at least 2 of the widely available testing modalities be used together.

Examples of well-known neurophysiological tests used in detecting brain dysfunction in patients with MHE are as follows:

Psychometric hepatic encephalopathy score: A paper and pencil test that has been reproduced and translated in many regions of the world.[61] This test can evaluate the speed at which specific cognitive tasks are performed.

Animal naming test: A neuropsychological bedside test that records the number of animals a patient can list within 60 seconds. This test also can predict the probability of progression from MHE to overt HE.[62]

Continuous reaction time (CRT): This is a computerized test that measures the stability of reaction times to an external stimulus. This measure is termed CRT index.[63] Additionally, the CRT test can determine if brain dysfunction has either a metabolic or an organic cause and the result is not affected by the patient's age or sex.[64]

Inhibitory control test: This is also a computerized test of response inhibition and working memory and is a test of good validity.[65]

Stroop test evaluates psychomotor speed and cognitive flexibility by the interference between recognition reaction time to a colored field and a written color name.[66]

Table 2	
West Haven criteria for semiquantitative grading of mental status[4]	
Grade	**Criteria**
1	Trivial lack of awareness Euphoria or anxiety Shortened attention span Impaired performance of addition
2	Lethargy or apathy Minimal disorientation of time or place Subtle personality changes Inappropriate behavior
3	Somnolence to semistupor but responsive to verbal stimuli Confusion Gross disorientation
4	Coma (unresponsive to verbal or noxious stimuli)

Electroencephalogram (EEG): This can detect alterations in cerebral cortical activity across the various forms of HE highlighted above; however, result can be affected by electrolyte abnormalities and medications.[59] The need for expert evaluation and interpretation of result and the varying cost of the procedures among hospitals may limit the use of EEG.

The critical flicker frequency (CFF): This test is a psychophysiological tool and is defined as the frequency at which a light seems to be flickering to an observer. This frequency is said to decrease with worsening cognition and seems to improve with treatment. This test requires repeated trials and specialized equipment.[67,68]

SUMMARY

In summary, the clinical presentation of HE in patients with acute and chronic liver disease manifests across a spectrum of severity, from early covert symptoms that may only be accurately detected with careful attention and specialized testing to overt symptoms that often accompany development of liver decompensation and/or liver failure. Greater awareness of the clinical manifestations, the different diagnostic modalities available for the assessment of presence and severity of HE allow timely identification, accurate assessment of HE severity grade, and ultimately help facilitate timely initiation of appropriate therapy.

CLINICS CARE POINTS

- Hepatic encephalopathy can occur in patients with acute liver failure as well as a complication of chronic liver disease and cirrhosis.
- Early recognition and timely diagnosis of hepatic encephalopathy is key to ensuring appropriate initiation of therapy to prevent associated morbidity and mortality.
- Several neurophysiological tests are available to evaluate the presence of hepatic encephalopathy, including psychometric hepatic encephalopathy score, animal naming test, continuous reaction time, inhibitory control test, stroop test, and the critical flicker frequency.

DISCLOSURE

No relevant disclosures for all authors.

REFERENCES

1. Wijdicks EF. Hepatic encephalopathy. N Engl J Med 2016;375(17):1660–70.
2. Ferenci P. Hepatic encephalopathy. Gastroenterol Rep (Oxf) 2017;5(2):138–47.
3. Vilstrup H, Amodio P, Bajaj J, et al. Hepatic encephalopathy in chronic liver disease: 2014 practice Guideline by the American association for the study of liver diseases and the European association for the study of the liver. Hepatology 2014;60(2):715–35.
4. Ferenci P, Lockwood A, Mullen K, et al. Hepatic encephalopathy–definition, nomenclature, diagnosis, and quantification: final report of the working party at the 11th World Congresses of Gastroenterology, Vienna, 1998. Hepatology 2002;35(3):716–21.
5. Louissaint J, Deutsch-Link S, Tapper EB. Changing epidemiology of cirrhosis and hepatic encephalopathy. Clin Gastroenterol Hepatol 2022;20(8S):S1–8.

6. Tapper EB, Henderson JB, Parikh ND, et al. Incidence of and risk factors for hepatic encephalopathy in a population-based cohort of Americans with cirrhosis. Hepatol Commun 2019;3(11):1510–9.
7. Orman ES, Roberts A, Ghabril M, et al. Trends in Characteristics, mortality, and other outcomes of patients with Newly diagnosed cirrhosis. JAMA Netw Open 2019;2(6):e196412.
8. Hirode G, Vittinghoff E, Wong RJ. Increasing burden of hepatic encephalopathy among hospitalized Adults: an analysis of the 2010-2014 national Inpatient sample. Dig Dis Sci 2019;64(6):1448–57.
9. Hirode G, Saab S, Wong RJ. Trends in the burden of chronic liver disease among hospitalized US Adults. JAMA Netw Open 2020;3(4):e201997.
10. Paik JM, Golabi P, Younossi Y, et al. Changes in the Global burden of chronic liver diseases from 2012 to 2017: the Growing impact of NAFLD. Hepatology 2020; 72(5):1605–16.
11. Younossi Z, Anstee QM, Marietti M, et al. Global burden of NAFLD and NASH: trends, predictions, risk factors and prevention. Nat Rev Gastroenterol Hepatol 2018;15(1):11–20.
12. Wong RKN, Meyer N, Gordon S. Rising and higher healthcare resource utilization (HCRU) and costs of Nonalcoholic Fatty Liver Disease (NAFLD)/Nonalcoholic Steatohepatitis (NASH) patients with advanced liver disease of increasing severity – Results of a US real-world analysis. Hepatology 2018;68(Suppl 1): 1284-1284A.
13. Wong RFN, Kent S, Gordon S. Significantly increased healthcare utilization and costs following diagnosis compensated cirrhosis among patients with nonalcoholic fatty liver disease and nonalcoholic steatohepatitis: real-world analysis of U.S. patients. Gastroenterology 2018;154(6):S-1110.
14. Wong RJ, Liu B, Bhuket T. Significant burden of nonalcoholic fatty liver disease with advanced fibrosis in the US: a cross-sectional analysis of 2011-2014 National Health and Nutrition Examination Survey. Alimentary pharmacology & therapeutics 2017;46(10):974–80.
15. Wong RJ, Singal AK. Trends in liver disease Etiology among Adults Awaiting liver transplantation in the United States, 2014-2019. JAMA Netw Open 2020;3(2): e1920294.
16. Singal AK, Arora S, Wong RJ, et al. Increasing burden of acute-on-chronic liver failure among alcohol-associated liver disease in the Young population in the United States. Am J Gastroenterol 2020;115(1):88–95.
17. Wong T, Dang K, Ladhani S, et al. Prevalence of alcoholic fatty liver disease among Adults in the United States, 2001-2016. JAMA 2019;321(17):1723–5.
18. Dang K, Hirode G, Singal AK, et al. Alcoholic liver disease epidemiology in the united states: a retrospective analysis of three United States databases. Am J Gastroenterol 2020;115(1):96–104.
19. Tapper EB, Parikh ND. Mortality due to cirrhosis and liver cancer in the United States, 1999-2016: observational study. Bmj 2018;362:k2817.
20. Long L, Li H, Deng G, et al. Impact of hepatic encephalopathy on clinical Characteristics and Adverse outcomes in prospective and multicenter Cohorts of patients with acute-on-chronic liver diseases. Front Med 2021;8:709884.
21. Labenz C, Nagel M, Kremer WM, et al. Association between diabetes mellitus and hepatic encephalopathy in patients with cirrhosis. Alimentary pharmacology & therapeutics 2020;52(3):527–36.
22. Jepsen P, Watson H, Andersen PK, et al. Diabetes as a risk factor for hepatic encephalopathy in cirrhosis patients. Journal of hepatology 2015;63(5):1133–8.

23. Nightingale JMD, Paine P, McLaughlin J, et al. The management of adult patients with severe chronic small intestinal dysmotility. Gut 2020;69(12):2074–92.
24. Patel VC, White H, Stoy S, et al. Clinical science workshop: targeting the gut-liver-brain axis. Metab Brain Dis 2016;31(6):1327–37.
25. Trebicka J, Macnaughtan J, Schnabl B, et al. The microbiota in cirrhosis and its role in hepatic decompensation. Journal of hepatology 2021;75(Suppl 1):S67–81.
26. Tapper EB, Jiang ZG, Patwardhan VR. Refining the ammonia hypothesis: a physiology-driven approach to the treatment of hepatic encephalopathy. Mayo Clin Proc 2015;90(5):646–58.
27. Cheon SY, Song J. The association between hepatic encephalopathy and diabetic encephalopathy: the brain-liver Axis. Int J Mol Sci 2021;22(1).
28. Agbalajobi OM, Gmelin T, Moon AM, et al. Characteristics of opioid prescribing to outpatients with chronic liver diseases: a call for action. PLoS One 2021;16(12): e0261377.
29. Moon AM, Jiang Y, Rogal SS, et al. Opioid prescriptions are associated with hepatic encephalopathy in a national cohort of patients with compensated cirrhosis. Alimentary pharmacology & therapeutics 2020;51(6):652–60.
30. Adams RD, Foley JM. The neurological disorder associated with liver disease. Res Publ Assoc Res Nerv Ment Dis 1953;32:198–237.
31. Seraj SM, Campbell EJ, Argyropoulos SK, et al. Hospital readmissions in decompensated cirrhotics: factors pointing toward a prevention strategy. World J Gastroenterol : WJG 2017;23(37):6868–76.
32. Rosenblatt R, Cohen-Mekelburg S, Shen N, et al. Cirrhosis as a Comorbidity in Conditions Subject to the hospital readmissions reduction Program. Am J Gastroenterol 2019;114(9):1488–95.
33. Gaspar R, Rodrigues S, Silva M, et al. Predictive models of mortality and hospital readmission of patients with decompensated liver cirrhosis. Dig Liver Dis 2019; 51(10):1423–9.
34. Yuan LT, Chuah SK, Yang SC, et al. Multiple bacterial infections increase the risk of hepatic encephalopathy in patients with cirrhosis. PLoS One 2018;13(5): e0197127.
35. Bajaj JS, Schubert CM, Heuman DM, et al. Persistence of cognitive impairment after resolution of overt hepatic encephalopathy. Gastroenterology 2010;138(7): 2332–40.
36. Callahan KE, Lovato JF, Miller ME, et al. Associations between mild cognitive impairment and hospitalization and readmission. J Am Geriatr Soc 2015;63(9): 1880–5.
37. Volk ML, Burne R, Guerin A, et al. Hospitalizations and healthcare costs associated with rifaximin versus lactulose treatment among commercially insured patients with hepatic encephalopathy in the United States. J Med Econ 2021; 24(1):202–11.
38. Bajaj JS, Reddy KR, Tandon P, et al. The 3-month readmission rate remains unacceptably high in a large North American cohort of patients with cirrhosis. Hepatology 2016;64(1):200–8.
39. Tapper EB, Essien UR, Zhao Z, et al. Racial and ethnic disparities in rifaximin use and subspecialty referrals for patients with hepatic encephalopathy in the United States. Journal of hepatology 2022;77(2):377–82.
40. Essien UR, Dusetzina SB, Gellad WF. A Policy prescription for reducing health disparities-Achieving pharmacoequity. JAMA 2021;326(18):1793–4.

41. Jesudian AB, Ahmad M, Bozkaya D, et al. Cost-effectiveness of rifaximin treatment in patients with hepatic encephalopathy. Journal of managed care & specialty pharmacy 2020;26(6):750–7.

42. Bernal W, Hyyrylainen A, Gera A, et al. Lessons from look-back in acute liver failure? A single centre experience of 3300 patients. Journal of hepatology 2013; 59(1):74–80.

43. Delanty N, French JA, Labar DR, et al. Status epilepticus arising de novo in hospitalized patients: an analysis of 41 patients. Seizure 2001;10(2):116–9.

44. Montagnese S, Turco M, Amodio P. Hepatic encephalopathy and sleepiness: an interesting connection? J Clin Exp Hepatol 2015;5(Suppl 1):S49–53.

45. Treem WR. Fulminant hepatic failure in children. J Pediatr Gastroenterol Nutr 2002;35(Suppl 1):S33–8.

46. Rodriguez-Rodriguez A, Egea-Guerrero JJ, Gordillo-Escobar E, et al. S100B and Neuron-Specific Enolase as mortality predictors in patients with severe traumatic brain injury. Neurol Res 2016;38(2):130–7.

47. Yardan T, Cevik Y, Donderici O, et al. Elevated serum S100B protein and neuron-specific enolase levels in carbon monoxide poisoning. The American journal of emergency medicine 2009;27(7):838–42.

48. Olivecrona Z, Bobinski L, Koskinen LO. Association of ICP, CPP, CT findings and S-100B and NSE in severe traumatic head injury. Prognostic value of the biomarkers. Brain Inj 2015;29(4):446–54.

49. Cordoba J, Cabrera J, Lataif L, et al. High prevalence of sleep disturbance in cirrhosis. Hepatology 1998;27(2):339–45.

50. Montagnese S, Middleton B, Skene DJ, et al. Night-time sleep disturbance does not correlate with neuropsychiatric impairment in patients with cirrhosis. Liver Int 2009;29(9):1372–82.

51. Mostacci B, Ferlisi M, Baldi Antognini A, et al. Sleep disturbance and daytime sleepiness in patients with cirrhosis: a case control study. Neurol Sci 2008; 29(4):237–40.

52. Amodio P, Montagnese S, Gatta A, et al. Characteristics of minimal hepatic encephalopathy. Metab Brain Dis 2004;19(3–4):253–67.

53. McCrea M, Cordoba J, Vessey G, et al. Neuropsychological characterization and detection of subclinical hepatic encephalopathy. Arch Neurol 1996;53(8):758–63.

54. The neuro-psychiatric syndrome associated with chronic liver disease and an extensive portal-systemic collateral circulation. Cent Afr J Med 1967;13(6):147.

55. Baccarani U, Zola E, Adani GL, et al. Reversal of hepatic myelopathy after liver transplantation: fifteen plus one. Liver Transplant 2010;16(11):1336–7.

56. Victor M, Adams RD, Cole M. The acquired (non-Wilsonian) type of chronic hepatocerebral degeneration. Medicine 1965;44(5):345–96.

57. Cordoba J, Ventura-Cots M, Simon-Talero M, et al. Characteristics, risk factors, and mortality of cirrhotic patients hospitalized for hepatic encephalopathy with and without acute-on-chronic liver failure (ACLF). Journal of hepatology 2014; 60(2):275–81.

58. Montagnese S, Amodio P, Morgan MY. Methods for diagnosing hepatic encephalopathy in patients with cirrhosis: a multidimensional approach. Metab Brain Dis 2004;19(3–4):281–312.

59. Guerit JM, Amantini A, Fischer C, et al. Neurophysiological investigations of hepatic encephalopathy: ISHEN practice guidelines. Liver Int : official journal of the International Association for the Study of the Liver 2009;29(6):789–96.

60. Randolph C, Hilsabeck R, Kato A, et al. Neuropsychological assessment of hepatic encephalopathy: ISHEN practice guidelines. Liver Int : official journal of the International Association for the Study of the Liver 2009;29(5):629–35.
61. Gabriel MM, Kircheis G, Hardtke S, et al. Risk of recurrent hepatic encephalopathy in patients with liver cirrhosis: a German registry study. Eur J Gastroenterol Hepatol 2021;33(9):1185–93.
62. Campagna F, Montagnese S, Ridola L, et al. The animal naming test: an easy tool for the assessment of hepatic encephalopathy. Hepatology 2017;66(1):198–208.
63. Lauridsen MM, Mikkelsen S, Svensson T, et al. The continuous reaction time test for minimal hepatic encephalopathy validated by a randomized controlled multimodal intervention-A pilot study. PLoS One 2017;12(10):e0185412.
64. Lauridsen MM, Thiele M, Kimer N, et al. The continuous reaction times method for diagnosing, grading, and monitoring minimal/covert hepatic encephalopathy. Metab Brain Dis 2013;28(2):231–4.
65. Bajaj JS, Hafeezullah M, Franco J, et al. Inhibitory control test for the diagnosis of minimal hepatic encephalopathy. Gastroenterology 2008;135(5):1591–600.e1.
66. Allampati S, Duarte-Rojo A, Thacker LR, et al. Diagnosis of minimal hepatic encephalopathy using Stroop EncephalApp: a multicenter US-based, Norm-based study. Am J Gastroenterol 2016;111(1):78–86.
67. Kircheis G, Wettstein M, Timmermann L, et al. Critical flicker frequency for quantification of low-grade hepatic encephalopathy. Hepatology 2002;35(2):357–66.
68. Romero-Gomez M, Cordoba J, Jover R, et al. Value of the critical flicker frequency in patients with minimal hepatic encephalopathy. Hepatology 2007;45(4):879–85.

The Health Care Burden of Hepatic Encephalopathy

Kevin B. Harris, MD[a], Humberto C. Gonzalez, MD[a,b],
Stuart C. Gordon, MD[a,b],*

KEYWORDS

- Hepatic • Encephalopathy • Cirrhosis • Liver transplantation • Liver disease • Cost

KEY POINTS

- Hepatic encephalopathy (HE) is a potentially reversible neurocognitive complication affecting approximately 30% of patients with cirrhosis.
- HE is responsible for tens of thousands of emergency department visits in the United States each year with an average cost of $2858 per visit. Total inpatient charges associated with HE exceed 10 billion US dollars per year.
- In addition to health care costs, HE creates a large economic burden due to missed work and inability to drive and operate heavy machinery.
- There are significant psychological and financial costs associated with being a primary caregiver for a patient with HE.

INTRODUCTION

Hepatic encephalopathy (HE) is a potentially reversible neurocognitive complication of liver cirrhosis. There are more than 600,000 adults in the United States living with cirrhosis,[1] with HE occurring among roughly 30% of cirrhotic patients.[2] HE can manifest with a spectrum of neurologic abnormalities, from subclinical changes to significant confusion and coma. It also increases morbidity and mortality associated with cirrhosis[3]; the survival probability after a first episode of HE is 42% at 1 year and 23% at 3 years.[4] In this article, the authors review the significant economic burden that HE imposes on caregivers and the US health care system.

PATHOPHYSIOLOGY OF HEPATIC ENCEPHALOPATHY

The pathophysiology of HE is complex and is an ongoing area of investigation. Liver dysfunction leads to a buildup of blood-derived products, which believes to alter

[a] Division of Gastroenterology and Hepatology, Henry Ford Health, Detroit, MI, USA; [b] Wayne State University, School of Medicine, Detroit, MI, USA
* Corresponding author. Henry Ford Hospital, 2799 W. Grand Boulevard, K16, Detroit, MI 48202.
E-mail address: sgordon3@hfhs.org

Clin Liver Dis 28 (2024) 265–272
https://doi.org/10.1016/j.cld.2024.01.009
1089-3261/24/© 2024 Elsevier Inc. All rights reserved.

the permeability of the blood-brain barrier.[3] Ammonia, bile acids, metals, and electrolyte imbalances all play integral roles in the development of HE.[3] Increased ammonia levels may lead to cellular swelling, oxidative stress, mitochondrial dysfunction, and changes in cell membrane potentials.[5] Emerging data also support a role for microbiota–host interactions in the pathogenesis of HE.[6] Treatment of HE includes treatment of acute episodes of HE and secondary prophylaxis for prevention of recurrence.[7] Reducing the economic burden of HE may also require more proactive screening for HE. At least one study showed that over half (53%) of a cohort of cirrhotic patients without overt HE had covert HE when administered a cognitive battery test, and those patients had a higher risk of overt HE, hospitalization, and death in adjusted analyses.[8]

EMERGENCY DEPARTMENT VISITS AND HOSPITAL ADMISSIONS

HE is responsible for tens of thousands of emergency department (ED) visits in the United States each year. Data from the Healthcare Cost and Utilization Project reveal that there were 57,578 ED visits for HE in 2014, with an average cost per visit of $2858.[9] Moreover, the vast majority of patients presenting to the ED with HE require admission for ongoing treatment.[9,10] Hospital admission increases the health care costs associated with an episode of HE.

It is estimated that HE accounts for 0.33% of all hospitalizations in the United States.[11] In 2014, there were 31,182 hospital admissions with HE, and from 2010 to 2014, total inpatient charges associated with HE increased by 46.0% (8.15 billion USD to 11.9 billion USD).[12] Despite reported declines in mortality and lengths of hospital stay for patients with decompensated cirrhosis from 2007 to 2017, related costs increased.[13] The average length of stay for patients hospitalized with HE decreased from 6.2 days to 4.9 days, but the average cost per admission increased from $38,897 to $49,391.[13]

Unfortunately, the economic costs associated with HE often do not end with the index admission. Approximately 22.2% of patients admitted with HE are discharged to nursing homes or rehab facilities, and another 16.2% are discharged with home health care services.[9] Skilled nursing facilities increase costs by an estimated $11,073, whereas home health services increase charges by an estimated $2,459.[14]

READMISSIONS

HE is a common reason for readmission for patients with decompensated cirrhosis,[15,16] accounting for 47% of readmissions for cirrhosis-related complications in one study.[17] In a single-center study of 402 cirrhotic patients, median time to readmission was 67 days, with 165 readmissions occurring within the first month after discharge.[18] Because HE readmissions are often costly, a substantial amount of quality improvement efforts have been devoted toward decreasing them. One quality improvement study that used electronic medical records (EMR) checklists to prompt providers to provide goal-directed lactulose therapy and rifaximin for patients with overt HE reported a 38% lower risk of readmission and decreased length of stay (−1.34) with use of the checklist.[19]

Another quality improvement initiative encouraged patients to use a mobile phone app known as a "patient buddy" to track clinical data and prevent readmission.[20] Participating patients and caregivers entered information on daily medication adherence, sodium intake, and body weight, along with weekly cognitive and fall risk assessments.[20] Of the 40 patients using the "patient buddy" app, 17 had readmissions within 30 days, but none of the readmissions were for HE.[20] Efforts have also been undertaken to better educate patients and caregivers on the pathophysiology of HE. One study examined the use of educational materials on patient outcomes.[21] One group of patients received educational materials on HE pathophysiology and medications and the importance of regular bowel movements in preventing episodes of encephalopathy.[21] Compared with standard of care, patients receiving the educational materials had a significant decrease in HE-related admissions (hazard ratio [HR] 0.14, CI 0.02 to 0.77).[21]

To improve transitions in care, some health systems have developed special post-discharge clinics for patients' admitted with HE.[22] For example, a group of patients with alcohol-related cirrhosis with HE were scheduled for follow-up at a specialty rehabilitation clinic before discharge; at the rehabilitation clinic, patients' clinical, psychological, and social issues were identified and addressed.[22] One-year survival was higher and alcohol consumption was lower in patients who followed up in the rehabilitation clinic compared with controls.[22]

Guidelines recommend lactulose as first-line therapy for HE and rifaximin in combination with lactulose for reducing the risk of HE recurrence.[7] Lactulose is a nonabsorbable disaccharide which acidifies the bowel milieu and increases intestinal transit and excretion of ammonia.[3] The dosing of lactulose is usually 15 to 20 mL titrated to 3 to 4 soft bowel movements per day.[3] Standard dosing of lactulose has been associated with a decrease in HE severity and mortality.[23] Unfortunately, the titratable nature of this medication can lead to lactulose ineffectiveness due to factors such as patient nonadherence or inadequate titration. Rifaximin is a non-aminoglycoside which acts against gram positive and gram negative aerobic and anaerobic enteric bacteria.[3] In a study of 299 patients who were in remission from recurrent HE, rifaximin significantly reduced the risk of an episode of HE when compared with placebo over a 6-month period (HR 0.42 95% CI 0.28–0.64).[24] Furthermore, in a double-blind randomized controlled trial, patients receiving lactulose and rifaximin had a shorter length of hospitalization (5.8 days vs 8.2 days) when compared with patients receiving lactulose alone.[25]

Inability to Work and Operate Heavy Machinery

In addition to the health care costs associated with HE hospitalizations, HE also creates a large economic burden due to missed work and disability claims. HE can impact job performance through decreased attention span, increased fatigue, and inability to operate work-related machinery. In a German study of 110 patients with cirrhosis, rates of HE were higher in blue-collar works (drivers, carpenters, factory workers) rather than white-collar workers (doctors, lawyers, academicians)[26]; 60% of blue-collar employees were deemed unfit for work by the German social security system compared with 20% of white-collar employees.[26]

One US study of 104 cirrhotic (44% with a history of HE) patients examined a variety of impacts of HE on patients' employment and personal finances.[27] Following the diagnosis of cirrhosis, 53% of patients decreased their work hours and 44% stopped working completely.[27] Patients with a history of HE had an unemployment rate of 87% compared with 19% in patients with no history of HE.[27] With decreased work hours, 56% of families stopped saving, 46% of families incurred debt, and 7% of families filed for bankruptcy.[27] The negative economic effects of HE may make it challenging for patients to afford medications and can lead to medication nonadherence.[27] This can create a cycle where medication nonadherence leads to hospital admissions, which increases the economic burden on patients and then promotes further nonadherence.

HE may impact the ability to safely drive and operate heavy machinery.[28] In a driving simulator study of 100 patients with cirrhosis and 67 controls, rates of collisions, speeding, and center line crossings were higher in patients with HE.[29] In addition, patients with HE were more likely to report fatigue after driving compared with controls.[29] Another study of 205 patients with cirrhosis categorized drivers as "safe" or "unsafe" based on crashes and violations reported on official driving records; 16% of patients with HE were characterized as unsafe compared with 7% of patients without HE.[30] Recognition of the deleterious effects HE can have on driver safety has led to recognition that hepatologists should ask patients with HE about driving safety and should recommend driving restrictions in patients with HE and prior poor driving history.[31,32]

Risks of Falls

In addition to increased risks of driving accidents, patients with HE are also prone to other injuries. Rates of falls are significantly higher in patients with cirrhosis and HE compared with patients with cirrhosis without cognitive issues.[33] Patients with cirrhosis who present to the ED with falls often have more severe injuries compared with patients without cirrhosis; rates of intracranial hemorrhage, skull fractures, and pelvic fractures are higher in patients with cirrhosis who present with falls.[34] The mean length of hospitalization for patients with cirrhosis following a fall is 7.25 days compared with 5.12 days in patients without cirrhosis.[34] Furthermore, the mean inpatient charges associated with a fall are higher in patients with cirrhosis ($61,808) compared with patients without cirrhosis ($43,106).[34]

Effects on Caregiver Quality of Life

In addition to the effects on patients themselves, there are significant psychological and financial costs associated with being a primary caregiver for a patient with HE. Caregivers report a sense of entrapment and a negative impact on their personal schedules and health compared with caregivers for patients without HE.[27] This is likely due to the detailed level of care required by patients with HE. In one study, 18% of care givers reported mild depression, 5% reported moderate depression, and 5% reported severe depression.[27] The patient's cognitive performance and model for end-stage liver disease (MELD) score were correlated with employment status and caregiver burden.[27] Patients with higher MELD scores and worse cognitive performance often require more detailed care making meaningful employment challenging and placing a larger psychological and financial strain on caregivers.

Treatment Options

Given the negative effects that HE has on quality of life for patients and caregivers, emphasis is placed on preventing and treating episodes of HE. Guidelines from the American Association for the Study of Liver Diseases (AASLD) recommend identifying and treating precipitating factors for HE, such as infections, GI bleeding, constipation, dehydration, and electrolyte derangements.[7] The AASLD also recommends therapies for HE including lactulose and rifaximin.[7] A recent meta-analysis of 16 studies demonstrated that lactulose and rifaximin improve several patient-reported outcomes in HE.[35] Lactulose and rifaximin also improved overall health-related quality of life, social activity, communication, and sleep in patients with HE.[35] A systematic review published in 2018 suggested the use of lactulose plus rifaximin reduces hospital readmissions and has a cost savings of $25–$49 million per year in the United States, compared with lactulose monotherapy.[36] There are increasing data that rifaximin is a cost-effective therapy for HE, both when used in conjunction with lactulose and used as a monotherapy. A large database analysis of 13,515 patients treated with rifaximin monotherapy and 9,946 patients with lactulose monotherapy revealed hospital admissions decreased by 33% when patients were treated with rifaximin versus lactulose alone.[37] Although higher pharmacy costs were associated with rifaximin, these costs were negated by the cost-saving effects on hospital admission rates and lengths of stay.[37] Similarly, a recent meta-analysis of 11 studies demonstrated rifaximin used as an add-on treatment with lactulose or as a monotherapy is a cost-effective treatment for HE when compared with lactulose alone.[38]

Despite the effectiveness of lactulose and rifaximin, HE continues to be a significant issue for patients with cirrhosis. A current research is focused on developing novel therapies for patients with HE. Enteric bacteria play a significant role in ammonia production; therefore, many future therapies for HE focus on altering gut bacteria composition.[6] Fecal microbial transplantation (FMT) has been proposed for treating HE.[39] In a study of patients with recurrent HE on lactulose plus rifaximin, 10 patients were randomized to receive FMT from the same donor, whereas 10 patients were randomized to receive standard of care.[40] No additional episodes of HE were experienced in the FMT group through 150 days compared with 6 episodes of HE in the standard of care group.[40] Further large-scale randomized studies are needed to evaluate the efficacy of FMT for patients with refractory HE. Studies have also investigated other novel therapies for HE including flumazenil, glycerol phenylbutyrate, L-ornithine L-aspartate, polyethylene glycol, and probiotics.[41] As our understanding of HE improves, it is likely novel therapeutic targets will continue to be identified.[41]

Role of Liver Transplantation

When considering the economic burden of HE, it is also important to consider costs associated with liver transplant, which is the definitive treatment of patients with decompensated cirrhosis. Although the presence of HE does not influence position on the transplant waitlist, the condition improves following liver transplantation, based on both cognitive function evaluations and neurologic imaging studies.[42] Costs associated with liver transplantation have risen substantially in the past decade, increasing from $577,100 in 2011 to $812,500 in 2017 (+41%).[43] Moreover, these numbers do not include the costs associated with the long-term immunosuppressive treatment that patients require posttransplant for the rest of their lives.

SUMMARY

As the prevalence of chronic liver disease increases throughout the United States, the health care burden of HE will continue to grow. HE results in direct health care costs through health care utilization and hospital admissions. Furthermore, HE creates indirect costs for patients and caregivers by affecting ability to work and quality of life. Current quality improvement initiatives are focused on improving transitions of care for patients with HE and decreasing hospital readmissions. There is also ongoing research focused on developing novel therapies for patients with refractory HE to improve quality of life for patients and caregivers. Continued efforts will be required to decrease the health care burden of HE.

CLINICS CARE POINTS

- Hepatic encephalopathy (HE) is a common complication of cirrhosis that affects survival and frequently results in hospital admissions.
- Beside the health care costs associated with hepatic encephalopathy, patients face economic burden from missed workdays and disability. Individuals with HE should be assessed for fall risk and driving safety.

- Identifying and treating precipitating factors for HE such as infections, GI bleeding and dehydration can shorten the duration of these episodes. Patients' and caregivers' education can reduce hospitalizations.

DISCLOSURE

No disclosures to report.

REFERENCES

1. Scaglione S, Kliethermes S, Cao G, et al. The epidemiology of cirrhosis in the United States: a population-based study. J Clin Gastroenterol 2015;49: 690–6.
2. Fallahzadeh MA, Rahimi RS. Hepatic encephalopathy: current and emerging treatment modalities. Clin Gastroenterol Hepatol 2022;20:S9–19.
3. Rose CF, Amodio P, Bajaj JS, et al. Hepatic encephalopathy: novel insights into classification, pathophysiology and therapy. J Hepatol 2020;73:1526–47.
4. Bustamante J, Rimola A, Ventura PJ, et al. Prognostic significance of hepatic encephalopathy in patients with cirrhosis. J Hepatol 1999;30:890–5.
5. Bosoi CR, Rose CF. Identifying the direct effects of ammonia on the brain. Metab Brain Dis 2009;24:95–102.
6. Bloom PP, Tapper EB, Young VB, et al. Microbiome therapeutics for hepatic encephalopathy. J Hepatol 2021;75:1452–64.
7. Vilstrup H, Amodio P, Bajaj J, et al. Hepatic encephalopathy in chronic liver disease: 2014 practice guideline by the American association for the study of liver diseases and the European association for the study of the liver. Hepatology 2014;60:715–35.
8. Patidar KR, Thacker LR, Wade JB, et al. Covert hepatic encephalopathy is independently associated with poor survival and increased risk of hospitalization. Am J Gastroenterol 2014;109:1757–63.
9. Elsaid MI, Rustgi VK. Epidemiology of hepatic encephalopathy. Clin Liver Dis 2020;24:157–74.
10. Ho CK, Maselli JH, Terrault NA, et al. High rate of hospital admissions among patients with cirrhosis seeking care in US emergency departments. Dig Dis Sci 2015;60:2183–9.
11. Stepanova M, Mishra A, Venkatesan C, et al. In-hospital mortality and economic burden associated with hepatic encephalopathy in the United States from 2005 to 2009. Clin Gastroenterol Hepatol 2012;10:1034–10341.e1.
12. Hirode G, Vittinghoff E, Wong RJ. Increasing burden of hepatic encephalopathy among hospitalized adults: an analysis of the 2010-2014 national inpatient sample. Dig Dis Sci 2019;64:1448–57.
13. Afridi F, Mittal A, Pyrsopoulos N. Trends in mortality and health care burden of cirrhotic decompensation in hospitalized patients: a nationwide analysis. J Clin Gastroenterol 2022;57:743–7.
14. Werner RM, Coe NB, Qi M, et al. Patient outcomes after hospital discharge to home with home health care vs to a skilled nursing facility. JAMA Intern Med 2019;179:617–23.
15. Bajaj JS, Reddy KR, Tandon P, et al. The 3-month readmission rate remains unacceptably high in a large North American cohort of patients with cirrhosis. Hepatology 2016;64:200–8.

16. Rosenstengle C, Kripalani S, Rahimi RS. Hepatic encephalopathy and strategies to prevent readmission from inadequate transitions of care. J Hosp Med 2022; 17(Suppl 1):S17–23.

17. Shaheen AA, Nguyen HH, Congly SE, et al. Nationwide estimates and risk factors of hospital readmission in patients with cirrhosis in the United States. Liver Int 2019;39:878–84.

18. Volk ML, Tocco RS, Bazick J, et al. Hospital readmissions among patients with decompensated cirrhosis. Am J Gastroenterol 2012;107:247–52.

19. Tapper EB, Finkelstein D, Mittleman MA, et al. A quality improvement initiative reduces 30-day rate of readmission for patients with cirrhosis. Clin Gastroenterol Hepatol 2016;14:753–9.

20. Ganapathy D, Acharya C, Lachar J, et al. The patient buddy app can potentially prevent hepatic encephalopathy-related readmissions. Liver Int 2017;37: 1843–51.

21. Garrido M, Turco M, Formentin C, et al. An educational tool for the prophylaxis of hepatic encephalopathy. BMJ Open Gastroenterol 2017;4:e000161.

22. Andersen MM, Aunt S, Jensen NM, et al. Rehabilitation for cirrhotic patients discharged after hepatic encephalopathy improves survival. Dan Med J 2013;60: A4683.

23. Gluud LL, Vilstrup H, Morgan MY. Non-absorbable disaccharides versus placebo/no intervention and lactulose versus lactitol for the prevention and treatment of hepatic encephalopathy in people with cirrhosis. Cochrane Database Syst Rev 2016;4:Cd003044.

24. Bass NM, Mullen KD, Sanyal A, et al. Rifaximin treatment in hepatic encephalopathy. N Engl J Med 2010;362:1071–81.

25. Sharma BC, Sharma P, Lunia MK, et al. A randomized, double-blind, controlled trial comparing rifaximin plus lactulose with lactulose alone in treatment of overt hepatic encephalopathy. Am J Gastroenterol 2013;108:1458–63.

26. Schomerus H, Hamster W. Quality of life in cirrhotics with minimal hepatic encephalopathy. Metab Brain Dis 2001;16:37–41.

27. Bajaj JS, Wade JB, Gibson DP, et al. The multi-dimensional burden of cirrhosis and hepatic encephalopathy on patients and caregivers. Am J Gastroenterol 2011;106:1646–53.

28. Reja M, Phelan LP, Senatore F, et al. Social impact of hepatic encephalopathy. Clin Liver Dis 2020;24:291–301.

29. Bajaj JS, Hafeezullah M, Zadvornova Y, et al. The effect of fatigue on driving skills in patients with hepatic encephalopathy. Am J Gastroenterol 2009;104:898–905.

30. Lauridsen MM, Thacker LR, White MB, et al. In patients with cirrhosis, driving simulator performance is associated with real-life driving. Clin Gastroenterol Hepatol 2016;14:747–52.

31. Lauridsen MM, Wade JB, Bajaj JS. What is the ethical (Not Legal) responsibility of a physician to treat minimal hepatic encephalopathy and advise patients not to drive? Clin Liver Dis 2015;6:86–9.

32. Tapper EB, Romero-Gómez M, Bajaj JS. Hepatic encephalopathy and traffic accidents: vigilance is needed. J Hepatol 2019;70:590–2.

33. Soriano G, Román E, Córdoba J, et al. Cognitive dysfunction in cirrhosis is associated with falls: a prospective study. Hepatology 2012;55:1922–30.

34. Ezaz G, Murphy SL, Mellinger J, et al. Increased morbidity and mortality associated with falls among patients with cirrhosis. Am J Med 2018;131:645–50.e2.

35. Moon AM, Kim HP, Jiang Y, et al. Systematic review and meta-analysis on the effects of lactulose and rifaximin on patient-reported outcomes in hepatic encephalopathy. Am J Gastroenterol 2023;118:284–93.

36. Neff G, Zachry W III. Systematic review of the economic burden of overt hepatic encephalopathy and pharmacoeconomic impact of rifaximin. Pharmacoeconomics 2018;36:809–22.

37. Volk ML, Burne R, Guérin A, et al. Hospitalizations and healthcare costs associated with rifaximin versus lactulose treatment among commercially insured patients with hepatic encephalopathy in the United States. J Med Econ 2021;24: 202–11.

38. Siddiqui KM, Attri S, Orlando M, et al. Cost-effectiveness of rifaximin-α versus lactulose for the treatment of recurrent episodes of overt hepatic encephalopathy: a meta-analysis. GastroHep 2022;2022:1298703.

39. Frenette CT, Levy C, Saab S. Hepatic encephalopathy-related hospitalizations in cirrhosis: transition of care and closing the revolving door. Dig Dis Sci 2022;67: 1994–2004.

40. Bajaj JS, Kassam Z, Fagan A, et al. Fecal microbiota transplant from a rational stool donor improves hepatic encephalopathy: a randomized clinical trial. Hepatology 2017;66:1727–38.

41. Alimirah M, Sadiq O, Gordon SC. Novel therapies in hepatic encephalopathy. Clin Liver Dis 2020;24:303–15.

42. Acharya C, Bajaj JS. Hepatic encephalopathy and liver transplantation: the past, present, and future toward equitable access. Liver Transplant 2021;27:1830–43.

43. Cook M, Zavala E. The finances of a liver transplant program. Curr Opin Organ Transplant 2019;24:156–60.

Social Impact of Hepatic Encephalopathy

Akshay Shetty, MD[a,b,*], Elena G. Saab[c], Gina Choi, MD[a,b]

KEYWORDS

- Hepatic encephalopathy • Cirrhosis • End-stage liver disease
- Health care utilization • Health care-related quality of life
- Driving and hepatic encephalopathy • Caregiver burden

KEY POINTS

- Hepatic encephalopathy (HE) leads to significant worsening in a patient's health-related quality of life and their ability to work. There is a growing need for point-of care standardized testing to diagnose minimal HE (MHE)/covert HE.
- Physicians should play an active role in patient education about the risks of driving in MHE patients, but the final authority for determination of driving fitness remains with each state's Department of Motor Vehicle agency.
- The burden on caregivers among cirrhosis and HE patients remains heavy, and early identification of stressors increasing risk of caregiver burden is crucial.

INTRODUCTION

Hepatic encephalopathy (HE) is among the most frequent decompensating events for patients with cirrhosis and associated with increased health care resource utilization.[1,2] Patients with HE suffer a wide spectrum of neurocognitive dysfunction, ranging from cognitive deficits, psychomotor slowing, mood changes, to disorientation and coma.[3] HE classification ideally includes the underlying etiology of liver disease, severity of HE manifestation, time course of the disease, and precipitating factors.[3] However, it can be broadly categorized into two divisions based on the severity of the disease: covert HE (CHE) and overt HE (OHE).[4] CHE is defined as the presence of neurocognitive dysfunction in patients, who are otherwise alert, oriented, and lack asterixis, and includes patients with minimal HE (MHE) and patients with grade 1 HE on the West Haven Criteria.[2,4]

Cirrhosis is the most common risk factor for HE, whose incidence has risen steadily over the last decade.[5] A reciprocal increase is expected in HE and its associated

[a] Department of Medicine, University of California at Los Angeles, Los Angeles, CA, USA;
[b] Department of Surgery, University of California at Los Angeles, Los Angeles, CA, USA;
[c] School of Medicine, Wake Forest University, Winston Salem, NC, USA
* Corresponding author. Pfleger Liver Institute, 100 Medical Plaza, Suite 700, Los Angeles, CA 90095.
E-mail address: akshayshetty@mednet.ucla.edu

Clin Liver Dis 28 (2024) 273–285
https://doi.org/10.1016/j.cld.2024.01.011
1089-3261/24/© 2024 Elsevier Inc. All rights reserved.

health care and societal costs. Among cirrhosis patients, cognitive dysfunction, presumed due to HE, led to the highest health care resource utilization compared with other manifestations.[1] Health-related quality of life (HRQoL) is significantly impaired among cirrhosis patients compared with healthy controls, with decompensated cirrhosis associated with worse HRQoL scores compared with compensated cirrhosis patients.[6] The presence of CHE and OHE are both associated with significant changes in a patient's quality of life (QoL), ability to work or drive, and caregiver burden (**Fig. 1**). In this review, the authors summarize the social impact of HE on patients and their caregivers.

QUALITY OF LIFE
Defining and Assessing Quality of Life

Medical outcomes have classically focused on morbidity and mortality related to a disease, but a shift in emphasizing the importance of a patient's QoL in relation to their disease is emerging, as QoL is gaining strength as an essential patient-centered outcome. HRQoL in cirrhosis patients is inversely associated to mortality and hospitalization rates, further highlighting its importance.[7,8] QoL is a multidimensional concept and is defined by the World Health Organizations as an individual's perception of their general well-being in terms of the physical, social, environmental, and cultural context.[9] Although QoL and HRQoL are routinely used interchangeably, QoL emphasizes a broader idea of patient's overall wellness compared with HRQoL, which focuses on the patient's perception on how a chronic illness impacts their QoL.[10] Measurement of HRQoL is a challenging task[11] and requires patients to complete questionnaires to study the impact of a chronic disease on different health domains, covering physical, mental, and social aspects.[12–17] Multiple questionnaires have been used in literature to assess HRQoL in patients with cirrhosis, and the authors have summarized the most commonly used questionnaires in **Table 1**. Among the six questionnaires included, only two are disease–specific, the Chronic Liver Disease Questionnaire (CLDQ) and Liver Disease Quality of Life 1.0 (LDQOL),[13,15] and were

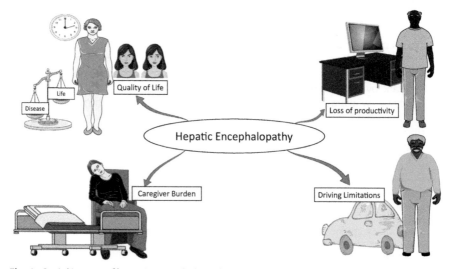

Fig. 1. Social impact of hepatic encephalopathy. (*Created by adapting and modifying* pictures from the "National Library of Medicine Image Resources. *Using free for use images under the Pixabay Content License. **The Figure was partly generated using Servier Medical Art, provided by Servier, licensed under a Creative Commons Attribution 3.0 unported license.).

Table 1
Quality of life assessment tools

Chronic Liver Disease Questionnaire	Liver Disease Quality of Life (LDQOL)	Nottingham Health Profile	Patient-Reported Outcomes Measurement Information System (PROMIS)	Short-Form Health Survey (SF-36)	Sickness Impact Profile
Abdominal symptoms	Part 1: SF-36	Part 1: Present distress	Anger	Bodily pain	Alertness behavior
Activity	Part 2: Disease-Targeted Supplement	Emotional reactions	Anxiety	Emotional role	Ambulation
Emotional function	Change in health over past 1 y	Energy	Depression	General health	Body care and movement
Fatigue symptoms	Concentration	Pain	Fatigue	Mental health	Communication
Systemic symptoms	Health distress	Physical mobility	Pain-behavior	Physical functioning	Eating
Worry	Hopelessness	Sleep	Pain-interference	Physical role	Emotional behavior
	Liver disease-related effects on activities of daily living	Social isolation	Physical function	Social functioning	Home management
	Liver disease-related symptoms	Part 2: Everyday activities	Satisfaction with discretionary social activities	Vitality	Mobility
	Loneliness	Employment	Satisfaction with social roles		Recreation and pastimes
	Memory	Hobbies	Sleep disturbance		Sleep and rest
	Quality of social interaction	Holidays	Sleep-related impairment		Social interactions
	Self-perceived stigma of liver disease	Home life			Work
	Sexual functioning	Household activities			
	Sexual problems	Sex life			
	Sleep	Social life			

designed for chronic liver disease patients, whereas the rest are intended for patients with general health conditions. Although there is no single best tool to assess HRQoL, each tool carries its own strengths and limitations. Experts suggest the use of disease-specific HRQoL tools in conjunction with generic questionnaires for optimal assessment.[18]

Hepatic Encephalopathy and Quality of Life

Conditions leading to cognitive deficits are negatively associated to a patient's QoL[19] and impact both patient and caregivers alike. Patients with cirrhosis complicated by HE are no exception to this, as noted in a recent single-center study of 246 cirrhosis patients in whom higher scores on global cognitive functioning testing, assessed by repeatable battery for the assessment of neuropsychological status (RBANS) and the Shipley Institute of Living Scale, were associated with higher HRQoL scores in both physical and mental health domains.[20]

Patients with overlapping symptoms in addition to MHE, such as depression or reduced appetite were noted to have worse HRQoL in comparison to non-MHE patients with similar such symptoms.[21–23] Overall, the presence of MHE and CHE have strongly been associated with poor HRQoL across several small and large studies.[8,20–33] A review of these studies, as summarized in **Table 2**, highlights the variability between studies in how the diagnosis of CHE or MHE was made and raises the need for standardized testing to diagnose MHE/CHE.

Despite the above links to poor HRQoL in HE patients, the authors may be under-reporting the impact that HE has on a patient's QoL. As discussed earlier, assessing HRQoL in general is a challenging task[11] and gets more difficult in HE patients with cognitive deficits. Measurement of HRQoL is conducted through questionnaires (see **Table 1**) requiring direct patient input, and thus by design, under represents patients with acute, episodic, or persistent OHE. Most of the studies also excluded patients with a prior history of OHE, as summarized in **Table 2**. Based on the impact that CHE or MHE has on QoL, one may extrapolate that OHE likely impacts QoL to a greater degree. In patients with a prior history of OHE that is currently well controlled, an Italian cohort suggested that prior history of OHE without active symptoms is still more likely to impair QoL than presence of MHE, further highlighting its significance.[31]

Although most of the studies have linked poor HRQoL to HE, some studies have argued against this association, in particular in patients with MHE. In a study of 87 patients with cirrhosis, where only 27 patients were diagnosed with MHE, MHE was not associated with changes in HRQoL based on short-form health survey (SF-36) and CLDQ questionnaires.[34] In a separate Danish cohort of 92 compensated cirrhosis patients, MHE was not associated with HRQoL, but the investigators questioned whether study size may have played a role.[35] Both studies had small sample sizes, raising questions about selection bias. Patients with MHE have been shown to have poor insight in to their multitasking abilities and may over estimate their self-reports on HRQoL questionnaires.[36] Second, cirrhosis itself is strongly associated with poor HRQoL, with sicker, decompensated cirrhosis patients having worse HRQoL scores compared with compensated cirrhosis or patients with chronic liver disease.[6] This raises the question of whether HRQoL is a function of progressive liver disease in addition to HE, rather than HE alone.

Impact of Hepatic Encephalopathy Treatment on Quality of Life

Treatment for HE has been associated with improvement in cognitive function among HE patients,[37] but limited number of studies have reviewed changes in HRQoL with

Table 2
Associations between hepatic encephalopathy and health-related quality of life

Author of Study	N = Patients (%HE)	History of OHE	HE Diagnosis Made by	HRQoL Surveys Used	HE Negatively Effects QoL
Groeneweg et al,[27] 1998	179 (26.8%)	N	NCT-A, DST	SIP	Y
Tan et al,[33] 2009	62 (33.9%)	N	NCT-A, DST, BDT	SIP	Y
Les et al,[30] 2010	212 (48%)	Y	TMT, SDT, GPT	SF-36, CLDQ	Y
Bajaj et al,[25] 2011	104 (44%)	Y	NS	PROMIS, SIP	Y
Wunsch et al,[34] 2011	77 (37.7%)	N	PHES	SF-36, CLDQ	N
Moscucci et al,[31] 2011	75 (42.7%)	Y	PHES, SPHES	SF-36	Y
Ahluwalia et al,[24] 2013	82 (51.2%)	Y	PHES	SIP	Y
Wang et al,[32] 2013	519 (39.9%)	N	NCT-A, DST	MC-QoL	Y
Nardelli et al,[23] 2013	60 (36.7%)	Y	PHES	SF-36	Y
Thiele et al,[35] 2013	92 (22.6%)	N	CRT	CLDQ	N
Mina et al,[21] 2014	125 (44.0%)	N	PHES	CLDQ	Y
Barboza et al,[22] 2016	43 (76.7%)	Y	NCT, D-KEFS, WAIS-III BDDSC	SF-36, LDQOL 1.0	Y
Paulson et al,[20] 2016	246 (NS)	NS	RBANS, TMT, SILS	SF-36	Y
Bajaj et al,[26] 2016	205 (40.5%)	Y	PHES	PROMIS	Y
Patidar et al,[8] 2017	286 (40%)	Y	Clinical history, HE medications	PROMIS	Y
Labenz et al,[28] 2018	145 (40.7%)	N	PHES, CFF	CLDQ	Y
Labenz et al,[29] 2019	139 (36.7%)	N	PHES, CFF	CLDQ	Y

Abbreviations: BDT, block design test; CFF, clicker flicker frequency; CLDQ, Chronic Liver Disease Questionnaire; CRT, continuous reaction time test; D-KEFS, Delis-Kaplan Executive Function System; DST, digit symbol test; GPT, Grooved Pegboard Test; HE, hepatic encephalopathy; HRQoL, health-related quality of life; LDQOL 1.0, Liver Disease Quality of Life Questionnaire; MC-QoL, Modified Chinese QoL questionnaire; NCT, number connection test; NCT-A, NCT Part A; N, No; NS, not specified; OHE, overt hepatic encephalopathy; PHES, psychometric hepatic encephalopathy score; PROMIS CAT, PROMIS computerized adaptive testing; PROMIS, patient-reported outcomes measurement information system; QoL, quality of life; RBANS, repeatable battery for the assessment of neuropsychological status; SDT, serial dotting test; SF-36, Medical Outcomes Study 36-item Short Form Health Survey; SILS, Shipley Institute of Living Scale; SIP, sickness impact profile; SPHES, simplified psychometric hepatic encephalopathy score; TMT, trail making test; WAIS-III BDDSC, Wechsler Adult Intelligence Scale 3rd Edition Block Design and Digit Symbol-Coding; Y, Yes.

treatment. In a non-blinded randomized control trial (RCT) of lactulose versus no treatment conducted in 61 patients with cirrhosis and MHE, 3 months of lactulose treatment led to improvement in neuropsychological test scores and HRQoL based on sickness impact profile (SIP).[38] Similarly, in an RCT of 160 patients with MHE and cirrhosis, 3 months of treatment with either lactulose, probiotics, or L-ornithine-L-aspartate led to improvement in HRQoL based on SIP in all groups compared with no treatment, with no difference seen when comparing each treatment head to head.[39] Probiotics were evaluated separately in an RCT of 30 patients, and compared with placebo, with no difference noted in HRQoL (SIP scores) after treatment.[40] Finally, rifaximin has been studied in MHE patients in two separate RCTs, and after 8 weeks of treatment, showed improvement but not a statistically significant change in HRQoL in the first study,[41] whereas the second study showed a statistically significant improvement in HRQoL after treatment.[42] Although the studies are limited, there is overwhelming evidence that treatment of HE leads to improvement in cognitive function, and therefore, reasonable to infer that improvement in HRQoL should be expected across all severities of HE.

LOSS OF PRODUCTIVITY AND WORKING CAPACITY

Employment plays a key role in a patient's QoL, where employed patients often rated their QoL approximately one-third of a standard deviation higher than unemployed patients.[43] HE diminishes cognitive function and a patient's ability to multitask, both crucial to employment in many fields. Although OHE has profound effects on cognition and psychomotor abilities, MHE patients have less pronounced changes with mild cognitive alterations effecting psychomotor function and practical intelligence, with preserved global cognitive ability.[44] Differences in cognitive abilities between OHE and MHE patients carry different implications for a patient's work capacity. Patients with a prior history of OHE have higher rates of unemployment compared with those without HE and notably worse financial status.[45] A review of unemployment status in patients with cirrhosis across three centers revealed higher rates of OHE in the unemployed group along with lower personal income than their employed counterparts.[46]

Meanwhile, MHE patients often have more subtle effects and are a major cause of premature retirement in cirrhosis patients.[44] The diminished practical intelligence and psychomotor functions in MHE disproportionally affect patients with professions that require motor coordination and attentiveness, such as drivers, skilled workers, craftsmen, or heavy machinery operators, often labeled as blue-collar jobs. In a German cohort of 110 cirrhosis patients, 60% of blue-collar workers were deemed unfit to work by a physician assessment based on the German social security parameters, whereas only 20% of white-collar workers were deemed unfit to work.[44] Although MHE was not directly assessed in the two groups, psychometric testing was surprisingly similar across both groups, with the exception of psychomotor function, which revealed that fitness to drive was worse in the non-working group.

Diminished work capacity related to HE carries significant socioeconomic impacts on a patient and their families, as the financial burden often falls on caregivers, leading to challenges in a patient's social support system. Unemployment among HE patients may disproportionately affect patients of lower socioeconomic status, who often have limited resources and carry higher financial insecurities.[45,46] Such challenges in a patient's finances combined with issues in social support systems may predispose patients to treatment nonadherence, inadvertently affecting their medical outcomes and potential liver transplantation candidacy.[47] Such risks may be mitigated by early discussions with patients and caregivers regarding the socioeconomic burden of liver disease in a multidisciplinary model, incorporating input from social workers, palliative care teams, financial officers, and hepatology.

DRIVING WITH HEPATIC ENCEPHALOPATHY

Motor vehicle crashes are preventable, but rates of crashes nationally in the United States continue to rise, and remain a leading cause of mortality.[48] Data from the US Department of Transportation (DOT) National Highway Traffic Safety Administration (NHTSA) reported a 6.8% increase in motor vehicle crash deaths from 2019 to 2020, despite an 11.0% drop in the number of miles traveled.[49] Motor vehicle crashes add to societal expense through both medical cost and patient related-mortality. Driving and navigating a motor vehicle requires complex coordination between spatial awareness, hand-eye coordination, and recall memory, often demanding instantaneous reaction times to make active decisions based on urgent current traffic cues.[47] Data from the NHTSA reported that driver error was the critical reason for motor vehicle accidents in 94% of crashes between 2005 and 2007.[50] Patients with MHE have deficits in the above areas, making driving quite dangerous for patients and for other drivers on the road. Early small studies provide conflicting results on MHEs association to a patient's driving abilities, with two studies[51,52] suggesting MHE patients were unfit to drive, whereas a Chicago case control of 15 patients with cirrhosis concluded no difference in driving ability based on real road driving between MHE and non-MHE patients.[53] Following these early studies, a larger German prospective study compared 48 cirrhosis patients to 49 controls patients where patients completed a standardized on-road driving test with a professional driving instructor and reported that MHE patients had lower driving scores compared with patients without MHE and controls.[50] In comparison to control and patients without MHE, the likelihood of a need for intervention to prevent an accident by the driving instructor was 10 times higher in the MHE patient group.

Recent studies using driving simulation tests compared 49 cirrhosis patients against 48 age- and education-matched control patients. Cirrhosis patients with MHE were noted to have impaired response inhibition leading to more illegal turns and higher number of accidents during the simulation test, correlating to poor navigational skills compared with cirrhosis patients without MHE and their matched controls.[54] Patients with MHE and prior history of OHE on therapy were also noted to be more susceptible to fatigue after similar driving simulations compared with non-MHE and age-/education-matched control patients, with fatigued patients at highest risk of accidents during simulations.[55]

Debate on whether all patients with MHE or only a specific subset of the MHE patients are at higher risk and should be deemed unfit to drive persists. Bajaj and colleagues[56] compared patients diagnosed with MHE based on paper–pencil standard psychometric tests (SPTs) to computerized inhibitor control test (ICT). ICT has been studied separately for MHE diagnosis and is associated with driving simulator performance.[54] Collision reports were collected for the patients with SPT-based MHE diagnosis and ICT-based MHE diagnosis from the year before diagnosis and the year after the diagnosis based on the patient self-reports and the DOT records. ICT-based MHE diagnosis patients were associated with significantly higher past and future collisions based on self- and DOT-reports compared with patients without MHE, whereas SPT-based MHE patients did not demonstrate a significant difference.[56] The duration of sobriety from alcohol use and presence of MHE has also been linked to real-life motor vehicle accidents and driving simulation navigation errors; of note, patients with less than 1 year of sobriety and MHE were more likely to get in to accidents.[57] Last, patients with MHE have poor insight into their driving capabilities and thus may not seek assistance from their caregivers, even when it is appropriate to do so. In a study of 47 cirrhosis patients and 40 control patients, MHE patients rated their driving skills to be equivalent to cirrhosis patients without MHE and the control patients despite having worse performance on driving simulator tests.[36] This highlights the importance of early diagnosis of MHE and the need for education to increase awareness of driving risks in this patient population. However, a blanket ban from driving for all patients with MHE may be too extreme, as a tailored approach to each patient's case based on prior driving records and current MHE diagnosis should be used. Future studies should focus on identifying optimal psychometric tests and risk factors that help categorize which MHE patients are at highest risk of driving errors. Driving simulation tests are not readily available at all centers, but when available, they should be used to assist in driving fitness assessment. Physicians should play an active role in patient education about the risks of driving in MHE patients, but the final authority for determination of driving fitness remains with each state's Department of Motor Vehicle agency.

CAREGIVER BURDEN

Informal caregivers, often composing of family members and friends, serve as the backbone for a patient's success through the management of their chronic medical conditions. In particular, caregivers are crucial to patients with cirrhosis and HE, especially if they are to be considered for liver transplantation.[58] Although care giving is rewarding, chronicity of HE is often characterized with high rates of hospitalizations and worsening cognitive function, which can take a significant toll on the caregivers. Caregiver burden is a complex multidimensional concept, impacting the physical, psychological, emotional, and financial domains of a caregiver.[59,60] Caregiver burden is often unrecognized due to a myriad of reasons, ranging from focus on the patient's comorbidities, insufficient training among providers to recognize it, and social stigmatization to self-care among caregivers to name a few. Cirrhosis, and in particular decompensated cirrhosis, is strongly associated with caregiver burden, with significant overlap noted in patients with HE among the decompensated cirrhosis patients.[61] History of OHE among patients with cirrhosis predicted greater likelihood of caregiver burden compared with patients without OHE, with significantly greater perceived burden among patients with greater severity of HE.[45,62,63] Caregivers of patients with MHE were also noted to have higher caregiver burden compared with patients without MHE.[63]

In assessment of psychological and emotional components, caregivers for patients with cirrhosis and episodic or persistent HE were noted to have a major psychological burden and led to impaired QoL.[62,64] In a cross-sectional study of 132 primary caregivers for patients with cirrhosis, history of HE notably predicted anxiety among caregivers based on the general anxiety disorder questionnaire.[62] Although HE has not yet been identified as a direct risk factor of depression among caregivers, depression is prevalent among caregivers of patients with cirrhosis and those awaiting liver transplantation.[62,65] Providers therefore need greater awareness to screen caregivers for burnout and underlying mental health conditions. In addition, lower socioeconomic status among cirrhosis patients has been linked to caregiver burden,[63] as treatment costs for cirrhosis patients have been associated with both depression and anxiety.[62] In patients with a prior history of HE, family income assessment revealed lower annual income and lower reserve assets compared with patients without a prior history of HE, but the difference did not reach statistical significance.[45] Although the difference in financial income was not statistically significant for patients with a history of HE, financial burden among caregivers of patients with chronic liver disease have led to an increase in depression and worsened perceived health among caregivers.[65–67]

Caregivers continue to play an essential role among patients with cirrhosis and HE, and their support is fundamental to a patient's liver transplant candidacy and successful posttransplant outcome. The burden on caregivers among cirrhosis and HE patients remains heavy, and early identification of stressors across all caregiver burden domains is crucial. Screening for mental health disorders among caregivers should be pursued routinely and professional services or ancillary support, based on each caregivers needs, should be provided. The early involvement of palliative care teams may help facilitate this process.

SUMMARY

HE patients suffer a wide spectrum of neurocognitive dysfunction, ranging from cognitive deficits and psychomotor slowing to coma. The incidence of cirrhosis has risen steadily over the last decade, with a reciprocal increase in HE and its associated health care and societal costs. The presence of CHE and OHE leads to significant changes in a patient's QoL, their ability to work and drive. HE therefore adds to the financial strain in patients and in turn making them more dependent on their caregivers. The chronicity of cirrhosis and HE leads to significant caregiver burden, often impacting their mental health and QoL. Thus, HE is correlated to multiple debilitating conditions that spread beyond the patient. Caregivers are crucial to patients with cirrhosis and HE, especially if they are to be considered for liver transplantation. There are unique challenges connected to cirrhosis and HE which compound its societal burden and warrant further understanding and study of this challenging group of patients.

CLINICS CARE POINTS

- Minimal or covert hepatic encephalopathy (HE) patients require a high index of suspicion to diagnose and early treatment should be promptly pursued.
- Quality of life assessments are often challenging to complete in decompensated cirrhosis patients, but may offer valuable information to help tailor patient care plans.

DISCLOSURE

Guarantor of article: A Shetty. Role in the Study: Study concept and design (A Shetty, G Choi); acquisition of data (A Shetty); analysis and interpretation of studies (A Shetty); drafting of the manuscript (A Shetty); critical revision of the manuscript for important intellectual content (A Shetty, G Choi); statistical analysis (N/A); obtained funding (N/A); administrative, technical, or material support (EG Saab); and study supervision (G Choi).

REFERENCES

1. Rakoski MO, McCammon RJ, Piette JD, et al. Burden of cirrhosis on older Americans and their families: analysis of the health and retirement study. Hepatology 2012;55(1):184–91.
2. Vilstrup H, Amodio P, Bajaj J, et al. Hepatic encephalopathy in chronic liver disease: 2014 practice guideline by the American association for the study of liver

diseases and the European association for the study of the liver. Hepatology 2014;60(2):715–35.

3. American Association for the Study of Liver Diseases, European Association for the Study of the Liver. Hepatic encephalopathy in chronic liver disease: 2014 practice guideline by the European association for the study of the liver and the American association for the study of liver diseases. J Hepatol 2014;61(3):642–59.

4. Patidar KR, Bajaj JS. Covert and overt hepatic encephalopathy: diagnosis and management. Clin Gastroenterol Hepatol 2015;13(12):2048–61.

5. Huang DQ, Terrault NA, Tacke F, et al. Global epidemiology of cirrhosis - aetiology, trends and predictions. Nat Rev Gastroenterol Hepatol 2023;20(6):388–98.

6. Peng JK, Hepgul N, Higginson IJ, et al. Symptom prevalence and quality of life of patients with end-stage liver disease: a systematic review and meta-analysis. Palliat Med 2019;33(1):24–36.

7. Kanwal F, Gralnek IM, Hays RD, et al. Health-related quality of life predicts mortality in patients with advanced chronic liver disease. Clin Gastroenterol Hepatol 2009;7(7):793–9.

8. Patidar KR, Thacker LR, Wade JB, et al. Symptom domain groups of the patient-reported outcomes measurement information system tools independently predict hospitalizations and Re-hospitalizations in cirrhosis. Dig Dis Sci 2017;62(5): 1173–9.

9. The Whoqol Group. The World Health Organization quality of life assessment (WHOQOL): development and general psychometric properties. Soc Sci Med 1998;46(12):1569–85.

10. Guyatt GH, Ferrans CE, Halyard MY, et al. Exploration of the value of health-related quality-of-life information from clinical research and into clinical practice. Mayo Clin Proc 2007;82(10):1229–39.

11. Buiting HM, Olthuis G. Importance of quality-of-life measurement throughout the disease course. JAMA Netw Open 2020;3(3):e200388.

12. Lins L, Carvalho FM. SF-36 total score as a single measure of health-related quality of life: scoping review. SAGE Open Med 2016;4. 2050312116671725.

13. Younossi ZM, Guyatt G, Kiwi M, et al. Development of a disease specific questionnaire to measure health related quality of life in patients with chronic liver disease. Gut 1999;45(2):295–300.

14. Bergner M, Bobbitt RA, Carter WB, et al. The Sickness Impact Profile: development and final revision of a health status measure. Med Care 1981;19(8): 787–805.

15. Gralnek IM, Hays RD, Kilbourne A, et al. Development and evaluation of the Liver Disease Quality of Life instrument in persons with advanced, chronic liver disease–the LDQOL 1.0. Am J Gastroenterol 2000;95(12):3552–65.

16. Hunt SM, McKenna SP, McEwen J, et al. A quantitative approach to perceived health status: a validation study. J Epidemiol Community Health 1980;34(4): 281–6.

17. Cella D, Yount S, Rothrock N, et al. The Patient-Reported Outcomes Measurement Information System (PROMIS): progress of an NIH Roadmap cooperative group during its first two years. Med Care 2007;45(5 Suppl 1):S3–11.

18. Loria A, Escheik C, Gerber NL, et al. Quality of life in cirrhosis. Curr Gastroenterol Rep 2013;15(1):301.

19. Stites SD, Harkins K, Rubright JD, et al. Relationships between cognitive complaints and quality of life in older adults with mild cognitive impairment, mild alzheimer disease dementia, and normal cognition. Alzheimer Dis Assoc Disord 2018;32(4):276–83.

20. Paulson D, Shah M, Miller-Matero LR, et al. Cognition predicts quality of life among patients with end-stage liver disease. Psychosomatics 2016;57(5): 514–21.

21. Mina A, Moran S, Ortiz-Olvera N, et al. Prevalence of minimal hepatic encephalopathy and quality of life in patients with decompensated cirrhosis. Hepatol Res 2014;44(10):E92–9.

22. Barboza KC, Salinas LM, Sahebjam F, et al. Impact of depressive symptoms and hepatic encephalopathy on health-related quality of life in cirrhotic hepatitis C patients. Metab Brain Dis 2016;31(4):869–80.

23. Nardelli S, Pentassuglio I, Pasquale C, et al. Depression, anxiety and alexithymia symptoms are major determinants of health related quality of life (HRQoL) in cirrhotic patients. Metab Brain Dis 2013;28(2):239–43.

24. Ahluwalia V, Wade JB, Thacker L, et al. Differential impact of hyponatremia and hepatic encephalopathy on health-related quality of life and brain metabolite abnormalities in cirrhosis. J Hepatol 2013;59(3):467–73.

25. Bajaj JS, Thacker LR, Wade JB, et al. PROMIS computerised adaptive tests are dynamic instruments to measure health-related quality of life in patients with cirrhosis. Aliment Pharmacol Ther 2011;34(9):1123–32.

26. Bajaj JS, White MB, Unser AB, et al. Cirrhotic patients have good insight into their daily functional impairment despite prior hepatic encephalopathy: comparison with PROMIS norms. Metab Brain Dis 2016;31(5):1199–203.

27. Groeneweg M, Quero JC, De Bruijn I, et al. Subclinical hepatic encephalopathy impairs daily functioning. Hepatology 1998;28(1):45–9.

28. Labenz C, Baron JS, Toenges G, et al. Prospective evaluation of the impact of covert hepatic encephalopathy on quality of life and sleep in cirrhotic patients. Aliment Pharmacol Ther 2018;48(3):313–21.

29. Labenz C, Toenges G, Schattenberg JM, et al. Clinical predictors for poor quality of life in patients with covert hepatic encephalopathy. J Clin Gastroenterol 2019; 53(7):e303–7.

30. Les I, Doval E, Flavià M, et al. Quality of life in cirrhosis is related to potentially treatable factors. Eur J Gastroenterol Hepatol 2010;22(2):221–7.

31. Moscucci F, Nardelli S, Pentassuglio I, et al. Previous overt hepatic encephalopathy rather than minimal hepatic encephalopathy impairs health-related quality of life in cirrhotic patients. Liver Int 2011;31(10):1505–10.

32. Wang JY, Zhang NP, Chi BR, et al. Prevalence of minimal hepatic encephalopathy and quality of life evaluations in hospitalized cirrhotic patients in China. World J Gastroenterol 2013;19(30):4984–91.

33. Tan HH, Lee GH, Thia KTJ, et al. Minimal hepatic encephalopathy runs a fluctuating course: results from a three-year prospective cohort follow-up study. Singap Med J 2009;50(3):255–60.

34. Wunsch E, Szymanik B, Post M, et al. Minimal hepatic encephalopathy does not impair health-related quality of life in patients with cirrhosis: a prospective study. Liver Int 2011;31(7):980–4.

35. Thiele M, Askgaard G, Timm HB, et al. Predictors of health-related quality of life in outpatients with cirrhosis: results from a prospective cohort. Hepat Res Treat 2013;2013:479639.

36. Bajaj JS, Saeian K, Hafeezullah M, et al. Patients with minimal hepatic encephalopathy have poor insight into their driving skills. Clin Gastroenterol Hepatol 2008; 6(10):1135–9 ; quiz 1065.

37. Gluud LL, Vilstrup H, Morgan MY. Non-absorbable disaccharides versus placebo/no intervention and lactulose versus lactitol for the prevention and treatment

of hepatic encephalopathy in people with cirrhosis. Cochrane Database Syst Rev 2016;2016(5):Cd003044.

38. Prasad S, Dhiman RK, Duseja A, et al. Lactulose improves cognitive functions and health-related quality of life in patients with cirrhosis who have minimal hepatic encephalopathy. Hepatology 2007;45(3):549–59.

39. Mittal VV, Sharma BC, Sharma P, et al. A randomized controlled trial comparing lactulose, probiotics, and L-ornithine L-aspartate in treatment of minimal hepatic encephalopathy. Eur J Gastroenterol Hepatol 2011;23(8):725–32.

40. Bajaj JS, Heuman DM, Hylemon PB, et al. Randomised clinical trial: lactobacillus GG modulates gut microbiome, metabolome and endotoxemia in patients with cirrhosis. Aliment Pharmacol Ther 2014;39(10):1113–25.

41. Bajaj JS, Heuman DM, Wade JB, et al. Rifaximin improves driving simulator performance in a randomized trial of patients with minimal hepatic encephalopathy. Gastroenterology 2011;140(2):478–87.e1.

42. Sidhu SS, Goyal O, Mishra BP, et al. Rifaximin improves psychometric performance and health-related quality of life in patients with minimal hepatic encephalopathy (the RIME Trial). Am J Gastroenterol 2011;106(2):307–16.

43. Pack TG, Szirony GM, Kushner JD, et al. Quality of life and employment in persons with multiple sclerosis. Work 2014;49(2):281–7.

44. Schomerus H, Hamster W. Quality of life in cirrhotics with minimal hepatic encephalopathy. Metab Brain Dis 2001;16(1–2):37–41.

45. Bajaj JS, Wade JB, Gibson DP, et al. The multi-dimensional burden of cirrhosis and hepatic encephalopathy on patients and caregivers. Am J Gastroenterol 2011;106(9):1646–53.

46. Bajaj JS, Riggio O, Allampati S, et al. Cognitive dysfunction is associated with poor socioeconomic status in patients with cirrhosis: an international multicenter study. Clin Gastroenterol Hepatol 2013;11(11):1511–6.

47. Stilley CS, DiMartini AF, de Vera ME, et al. Individual and environmental correlates and predictors of early adherence and outcomes after liver transplantation. Prog Transplant 2010;20(1):58–66 ; quiz 67.

48. Yellman MA S-SE, Sauber-Schatz EK. Otor vehicle crash deaths — United States and 28 other high-income countries, 2015 and 2019. MMWR (Morb Mortal Wkly Rep) 2022;71(26):837–43.

49. Administration, N.H.T.S.. Traffic safety facts—early estimate of motor vehicle traffic fatalities in 2021. Washington, DC: US Department of Transportation, National Highway Traffic Safety Administration; 2022.

50. Wein C, Koch H, Popp B, et al. Minimal hepatic encephalopathy impairs fitness to drive. Hepatology 2004;39(3):739–45.

51. Schomerus H, Hamster W, Blunck H, et al. Latent portasystemic encephalopathy. I. Nature of cerebral functional defects and their effect on fitness to drive. Dig Dis Sci 1981;26(7):622–30.

52. Watanabe A, Tuchida T, Yata Y, et al. Evaluation of neuropsychological function in patients with liver cirrhosis with special reference to their driving ability. Metab Brain Dis 1995;10(3):239–48.

53. Srivastava A, Mehta R, Rothke SP, et al. Fitness to drive in patients with cirrhosis and portal-systemic shunting: a pilot study evaluating driving performance. J Hepatol 1994;21(6):1023–8.

54. Bajaj JS, Hafeezullah M, Hoffmann RG, et al. Navigation skill impairment: another dimension of the driving difficulties in minimal hepatic encephalopathy. Hepatology 2008;47(2):596–604.

55. Bajaj JS, Hafeezullah M, Zadvornova Y, et al. The effect of fatigue on driving skills in patients with hepatic encephalopathy. Am J Gastroenterol 2009;104(4): 898–905.
56. Bajaj JS, Saeian K, Schubert CM, et al. Minimal hepatic encephalopathy is associated with motor vehicle crashes: the reality beyond the driving test. Hepatology 2009;50(4):1175–83.
57. Lauridsen MM, Thacker LR, White MB, et al. In Patients with cirrhosis, driving simulator performance is associated with real-life driving. Clin Gastroenterol Hepatol 2016;14(5):747–52.
58. Martin P, DiMartini A, Feng S, et al. Evaluation for liver transplantation in adults: 2013 practice guideline by the American association for the study of liver diseases and the American society of transplantation. Hepatology 2014;59(3): 1144–65.
59. Dang S, Badiye A, Kelkar G. The dementia caregiver–a primary care approach. South Med J 2008;101(12):1246–51.
60. Parks SM, Novielli KD. A practical guide to caring for caregivers. Am Fam Physician 2000;62(12):2613–22.
61. Donlan J, Ufere NN, Indriolo T, et al. Patient and caregiver perspectives on palliative care in end-stage liver disease. J Palliat Med 2021;24(5):719–24.
62. Hareendran A, Devadas K, Sreesh S, et al. Quality of life, caregiver burden and mental health disorders in primary caregivers of patients with Cirrhosis. Liver Int 2020;40(12):2939–49.
63. Shrestha D, Rathi S, Grover S, et al. Factors affecting psychological burden on the informal caregiver of patients with cirrhosis: looking beyond the patient. J Clin Exp Hepatol 2020;10(1):9–16.
64. Fabrellas N, Moreira R, Carol M, et al. Psychological burden of hepatic encephalopathy on patients and caregivers. Clin Transl Gastroenterol 2020;11(4): e00159.
65. Miyazaki ET, Dos Santos R, Miyazaki MC, et al. Patients on the waiting list for liver transplantation: caregiver burden and stress. Liver Transpl 2010;16(10):1164–8.
66. Bolkhir A, Loiselle MM, Evon DM, et al. Depression in primary caregivers of patients listed for liver or kidney transplantation. Prog Transplant 2007;17(3):193–8.
67. Cohen M, Katz D, Baruch Y. Stress among the family caregivers of liver transplant recipients. Prog Transplant 2007;17(1):48–53.

Pharmacologic Management of Hepatic Encephalopathy

Ali Khalessi, MD, Nikolaos T. Pyrsopoulos, MD, PhD, MBA, AGAF, FRCP*

KEYWORDS

- Hepatic encephalopathy • Nonabsorbable disaccharides • Lactulose • Rifaximin

KEY POINTS

- Hepatic encephalopathy pharmacologic management.
- Mechanism of therapies for hepatic encephalopathy.
- Hepatic encephalopathy first-line therapies.
- Hepatic encephalopathy second-line therapies.

INTRODUCTION

Medical management of the patient with hepatic encephalopathy first relies on several key principles of appropriate supportive care. This includes appropriate triage of patients based on the grade of hepatic encephalopathy to outpatient therapy, inpatient therapy, or intensive care unit (ICU) for closer monitoring and airway management. Additionally, reversal of common precipitants such as bleeding, infection, volume depletion, and renal failure is vital to ensuring increased efficacy of any of the below treatments. The first step for any patient with hepatic encephalopathy is to tailor management according to the ABCs of hepatic encephalopathy (ie, acute liver failure or portosystemic shunting or acute on chronic liver failure and cirrhosis). However, in terms of pharmacologic therapy, patients with overt hepatic encephalopathy have been shown to benefit from a rather restrictive number of pharmacologic therapies.

ELECTROLYTE DISTURBANCES, HYPOKALEMIA

Management of hypokalemia is essential for successful treatment of hepatic encephalopathy. It has been long hypothesized that potassium depletion increases serum ammonia and therefore the risk of overt hepatic encephalopathy. In 1962, Baertl and colleagues demonstrated that a diuretic regimen in patients with cirrhosis led to an increase in serum ammonia, with subsequent development of hepatic encephalopathy. Other studies from the 1950s and 1960s demonstrated similar results.[1] The

Rutgers New Jersey School of Medicine, 185 South Orange Avenue, MSB H-538, Newark, NJ 07103, USA
* Corresponding author.
E-mail address: pyrsopni@njms.rutgers.edu

Clin Liver Dis 28 (2024) 287–296
https://doi.org/10.1016/j.cld.2024.01.006
1089-3261/24/

proposed mechanism behind this association is renal metabolism of glutamine to enable recovery of potassium within the proximal tubule, a process that produces ammonium as a byproduct. In fact, studies have shown that hypokalemia is associated with longer ICU stays, higher mortality, and increased severity of hepatic encephalopathy.[2] Ullah and colleagues' cross-sectional study of 5000 patients with hepatic encephalopathy revealed a direct association with the degree of hypokalemia and the grading of hepatic encephalopathy, with 60% of patients with serum potassium less than 2.5 mEq/L being diagnosed with grade 4 hepatic encephalopathy, compared with 6.4% of patients with serum potassium greater than 3.4 mEq/L.[3] However, given the lack of available randomized controlled trial (RCT) evaluation of potassium supplementation and hepatic encephalopathy resolution, it remains unclear whether hypokalemia directly increases severity of hepatic encephalopathy, or that it is a prognostic marker for worsening decompensation. Regardless, given the available data supporting the physiologic mechanism linking hypokalemia to increased serum ammonia levels, it is reasonable to recommend potassium supplementation for correction of hypokalemia in hospitalized patients with overt hepatic encephalopathy.

NONABSORBABLE DISACCHARIDES

In general, the mainstay of traditional pharmacologic therapy for hepatic encephalopathy is aimed at lowering serum ammonia concentration. Of the available treatments, nonabsorbable disaccharides such as lactulose (a disaccharide of fructose and galactose) and lactitol have remained the most easily accessible and commonly used treatment modalities. Lactulose is inexpensive, readily available across most institutions, associated with only mild gastrointestinal side effects and is available in both an oral and rectal formulation should the patient be unable to tolerate oral medications. Lactulose and lactitol exert their effect on serum ammonia via multiple proposed mechanisms. It is believed the primary mechanism is the reduction of stool pH by lactulose, which favors the conversion of ammonia to ammonium, trapping it in the colonic membrane and instead promoting its utilization of its nitrogen for protein synthesis by the colonic flora. This reduction in pH is also thought to favor the destruction of urease producing bacteria, further reducing ammonia production via changes in the microbiota. An additional potential mechanism includes the laxative effect produced by the metabolism of sugars by colonic bacteria, reducing transit time and thus ammonia absorption (**Fig. 1**).[4] A typical effective dose to achieve these effects is 20 to 30 mg of lactulose every 2 hours, titrated to achieve 2 to 3 soft stools per day.

In 1969 Elkington and colleagues' small RCT demonstrated such a reduction in stool pH and ammonia concentration as well as improvements in electroencephalogram readings among patients receiving lactulose therapy compared with those receiving sorbitol.[5] Since then, numerous other studies, including a 2016 Cochrane review of 38 RCTs of 1828 patients have demonstrated similar beneficial responses of lactulose compared with placebo (relative risk [RR], 0.58; 95% CI, 0.50–0.69) among most patients with overt hepatic encephalopathy.[6] A more recent 2020 systemic review and meta-analysis of 1563 patients, when comparing lactulose to placebo, showed improved reversal of minimal hepatic encephalopathy (odds ratio [OR], 5.39; 95% prediction interval [PrI], 3.6–8.0; surface under the cumulative ranking curve [SUCRA], 67.2%; moderate quality) as well as prevention of overt hepatic encephalopathy (OR, 0.22; 95% PrI, 0.09–0.52; SUCRA, 73.9%; moderate quality).[7] However, it is important to note that during the several decades since its widespread use, large, rigorous, well-designed RCTs are limited, and so the evidence for nonabsorbable disaccharides is derived mostly from such systematic reviews. Despite these limitations

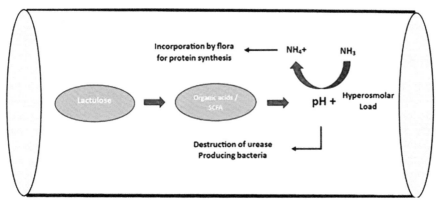

Fig. 1. Proposed mechanism of lactulose. Breakdown of lactulose by colonic bacteria produce short-chain fatty acids and other organic acids, reducing stool pH. This reduction in stool pH converts ammonia to ammonium, trapping it inside the colonic lumen and making it available for incorporation by the colonic flora into proteins. Additional mechanisms include the destruction of urease-producing bacteria by the reduction in stool pH, as well as an increase in hyperosmolar load via the production of organic acids, which then leads to a laxative effect, eliminating ammonia from the body.

in the available literature, lactulose remains the preferred first-line therapy for hepatic encephalopathy, partly because of its low price and thus high cost-effectiveness.[8]

Furthermore, RCTs by Sharma and colleagues and Agrawal and colleagues have demonstrated similar beneficial effects in the secondary prophylaxis of hepatic encephalopathy. Sharma and colleagues demonstrated a reduction in subsequent episodes from 47% with placebo to 20% with lactulose.[9,10] For this reason, both the American Association for the Study of Liver Diseases (AASLD) and European Association for the Study of the Liver (EASL) recommend continued use of lactulose after an initial episode of overt hepatic encephalopathy for secondary prophylaxis. Dosing remains similar to what is given for the reversal of overt symptoms.

POLYETHYLENE GLYCOL

If one of the mechanisms by which nonabsorbable disaccharides reduce serum ammonia is via a laxative effect, then it would be reasonable to hypothesize that other laxatives may be equally as efficacious. The 2014 HELP randomized clinical trial separated 50 patients with hepatic encephalopathy into either standard treatment with lactulose or treatment with 4 L of polyethylene glycol. Patients receiving polyethylene glycol saw resolution in hepatic encephalopathy at a median of 1 day, compared with 2 days for standard therapy with lactulose.[11] A 2021 systemic review and meta-analysis looked at studies similar to the HELP trial, for a total of 4 trials with 229 patients. The authors found that patients treated with polyethylene glycol scored lower on the hepatic encephalopathy scoring algorithm at 24 hours (mean difference, -0.68; CI, -1.05 to -0.31) were more likely to have a score of 0 at 24 hours (RR, -4.33; CI, 2.27–8.28) and have an overall shorter time to resolution of hepatic encephalopathy (MD, -1.45; CI, -1.72 to -1.18).[12] Despite the promising results so far for polyethylene glycol, evidence remains much sparser than that favoring treatment with lactulose. Additionally, the large volume required for treatment may not be effective in patients who are altered and may be higher aspiration risks. Whether there remains a role for polyethylene glycol in patients either unable to tolerate lactulose or have enteral access allowing easier administration of the 4 L required remains to be seen.

ANTIBIOTICS

Antibiotics to reduce serum ammonia concentrations have an established role in hepatic encephalopathy treatment. For many years neomycin, a glutaminase inhibitor, was the antibiotic of choice in reducing the burden of ammonia-producing bacteria. Early studies comparing neomycin and lactulose showed promising results, with several studies suggesting almost equal efficacy between the 2 treatments.[13] However, other subsequent studies were conflicting in their results. As an example, a randomized clinical trial of 102 cirrhotic patients with hepatic encephalopathy during hospital admission did not find a significant difference in resolution between patients receiving neomycin and those receiving placebo.[14] Additionally, neomycin has been repeatedly associated with significant adverse effects, including ototoxicity, nephrotoxicity, and neurotoxicity.[15] Evidence for other antibiotics, such as metronidazole, is even more lacking.

Several earlier studies have demonstrated promising results for rifaximin, a minimally absorbed oral antibiotic with both anaerobic and aerobic coverage of several gram positive and gram-negative bacteria. It is hypothesized that rifaximin works by altering the gut microbiota composition and enhancing the function of "positive microbiota" while also reducing the production of proinflammatory cytokines, although robust evidence for these hypotheses remains lacking.[16] A typical dose for rifaximin after an episode of hepatic encephalopathy is 550 mg twice daily for at least 3 months.

In 2003, an RCT of 103 patients by Mas and colleagues comparing lactitol with rifaximin demonstrated equal efficacy in the treatment of overt hepatic encephalopathy (81.6% vs 80.4%).[17] Since then, several more studies have demonstrated more promising results when comparing rifaximin against various other treatments for hepatic encephalopathy. In a subsequent 2013 RCT of 120 patients by Sharma and colleagues, the combination of lactulose and rifaximin proved superior to lactulose alone in the reversal of overt hepatic encephalopathy (76% vs 50.8%).[8] A 2014 systematic review by Kimer and colleagues demonstrated equal or greater efficacy for rifaximin with increased recovery from overt encephalopathy (RR, 0.59; CI, 0.46–0.76) and reduced mortality (RR, 0.68; CI, 0.48–0.97) when compared with lactulose, neomycin, and other antibiotics such as metronidazole. Overall, the number needed to treat was 4 when placebo controlled, 7 when lactulose controlled, and 6 when other antibiotics were used as the control.[18]

In terms of secondary prophylaxis, a 2010 RCT of 299 patients with a recent episode of hepatic encephalopathy found that rifaximin reduced the risk of a subsequent episode from 46% to 22% at 6 months,[19] with other studies demonstrating similar results. For this reason, most practitioners will use rifaximin in conjunction with lactulose for the prevention of overt hepatic encephalopathy in patients who have had a breakthrough episode while on lactulose. This practice is in line with both AASLD and EASL guidelines for the secondary prophylaxis of hepatic encephalopathy.

One of the drawbacks of rifaximin is its water-insolubility and dependence on bile acids for maximum effectiveness. In patients with liver disease microbiota dysbiosis resulting in bile acid imbalances may therefore reduce the effectiveness of rifaximin. More recently, a new soluble solid dispersion form of the medication has demonstrated increased water solubility with minimal system exposure and is available in both an immediate release and sustained release preparation. In a 2023 phase II clinical trial of 71 patients with overt hepatic encephalopathy, the immediate release version of this new formulation, when added to lactulose, reduced the median time to resolution of hepatic encephalopathy from 62.7 hours to 21.1 hours, when compared with lactulose alone.[20]

For these reasons, rifaximin, now approved by the Food and Drug Administration for treatment of hepatic encephalopathy, has largely overtaken other antibiotics such as neomycin and metronidazole. However, given the lower cost and ease of access with lactulose, rifaximin is used primarily as an adjunct to lactulose. Although some studies suggest that given its lower side-effect profile, the increased rate of adherence to rifaximin compared with lactulose may prevent hospitalizations for hepatic encephalopathy and thus make it perhaps even more cost-effective than lactulose, the available evidence is not strong enough to suggest a transition to rifaximin as the first-line therapy.[9] However, in patients who cannot tolerate lactulose due to its gastrointestinal side effects, rifaximin monotherapy may be a reasonable choice.

ALBUMIN

Albumin has seen widespread use among patients with decompensated cirrhosis, primarily for volume expansion and the treatment of hepatorenal syndrome. More recently, it has also been investigated as a potential pharmacologic therapy in the treatment of hepatic encephalopathy. Specifically, it is hypothesized that albumin infusions may reduce the level of proinflammatory cytokines as well as endothelial dysfunction, both of which may play a part in the precipitation of overt hepatic encephalopathy. This would allow for a therapeutic target separate from ammonia production and thus supplement the effect of the previously mentioned therapies.

A 2013 randomized control trial by Simon-Talero and colleagues assigned a total of 56 patients with grade II to IV hepatic encephalopathy to either receiving albumin with lactulose or saline with lactulose. Although there were no significant differences in hepatic encephalopathy at day 4, by day 90 there was a significant difference in survival favoring patients who received albumin (69.2% vs 40.0%). However, the authors admit that this difference in survival may have been that hepatic encephalopathy identifies more severely decompensated patients who may benefit from the anti-inflammatory properties of albumin.[21] A 2021 meta-analysis examined a total of 12 studies, with 2087 patients, and found that among patients with over hepatic encephalopathy, albumin infusion resulted in a lower overall risk (OR, 0.43; CI, 0.27–0.68). Furthermore, they also found a lower risk of developing overt hepatic encephalopathy in patients without any overt symptoms at baseline (OR, 0.53; CI, 0.32–0.86).[22]

Most recently, a 2023 double-blind randomized placebo-controlled trial by Fagan and colleagues, the HEAL study, looked at the impact of albumin on the prevention of hepatic encephalopathy. A total of 48 patients with prior hepatic encephalopathy or minimal hepatic encephalopathy despite treatment with standard of care were either treated with 25% IV albumin 1.5 g/kg or saline for 5 weeks. At 1 week after the last infusion, patients who received albumin had improvements in minimal hepatic encephalopathy scores, increased quality of life, and decreased endothelial dysfunction and inflammation interleukin 1 beta (IL-1B).[23] Although more studies are needed, this study and previous meta-analyses seem to indicate that there may be a role for albumin administration in patients with residual cognitive dysfunction despite treatment with standard of care.

BRANCHED-CHAIN AMINO ACIDS

It was previously thought that decreasing protein intake in patients with cirrhosis would decrease sources of nitrogen and thus serum ammonia levels and risk of overt hepatic encephalopathy. This has since been proven to be false, and it is instead now suggested to maintain a protein intake of at least 1.2 to 1.5 g/kg/d given the level of sarcopenia evident in most patients with cirrhosis. However, there does seem to be a subset of patients in whom protein intake is related to increase in serum ammonia. Among these patients, substitution of fish, milk, and meat protein with vegetable protein is thought to ameliorate this increase. This is thought to be due to not just the amino acid composition of vegetable proteins themselves but also the presence of fiber, which contains some level of nonabsorbable disaccharides.[24]

Another alternative to fish, milk, and meat protein is the administration of branched-chain amino acids. A 2015 cochrane review examined a total of 16 RCTs with 827 patients with overt or minimal hepatic encephalopathy confirmed a beneficial effect on branched-chain amino acids on hepatic encephalopathy (RR, 0.73; CI, 0.61–0.88). However, analysis of trials that compared branched-chain amino acids to lactulose or neomycin rather than placebo or just diet found no benefit (RR, 0.66; CI, 0.34–1.30).[25] The overall available evidence of branched-chain amino acids remains weak, although there does seem to be some role for supplementation in patients who are unable to tolerate protein intake or have no enteral access for nutritional support.

PROBIOTICS

The use of prebiotics such as nonabsorbable disaccharides may exert some of their clinical benefit via alterations in the gut microbiome. Therefore, it would not be unreasonable to assume that probiotic therapy may also play a role in the treatment of hepatic encephalopathy. A small 2008 randomized trial of 25 patients receiving a probiotic yogurt demonstrated significant reversal in minimal hepatic encephalopathy (71% vs 0%) and a reduction in the development of overt hepatic encephalopathy (0% vs 25%).[26] A 2017 meta-analysis of 21 trials with 1420 patients looked at the effectiveness of probiotics when compared with either placebo or lactulose. When compared with placebo, there was no effect on mortality but there was a lower rate of "no-recovery" (RR, 0.67; confidence interval [CI], 0.56–0.79) and a decrease in plasma ammonia (MD, -8.29 μmol/L; CI, -13.17 to -3.41). However, when compared with lactulose, these beneficial effects disappeared.[27]

A 2014 RCT of 160 patients by Lunia and colleagues looking specifically at the prevention of hepatic encephalopathy found that patients receiving probiotics, when compared with placebo, were less likely to develop overt HE (hazard ratio [HR], 2.1; CI, 1.31–6.53) and were also noted to have reduced levels of arterial ammonia.[28] Other studies looking at secondary prophylaxis have found similar results, although when compared with lactulose the benefit does not seem to be statistically significant.[10] Despite the significant limitations in studies looking at probiotics, especially since any systemic review or meta-analysis is likely to combine various forms or probiotics, there is promising data at least for the prevention of overt hepatic encephalopathy, if not for its treatment. More data are needed on the impact of specific microbes on overall ammonia balance before more promising trials can be conducted.

The current available data for the use of fecal microbiota transplant as a potential therapy for hepatic encephalopathy are even more limited than that of probiotics. A small 2017 open-label RCT of 28 patients with recurrent hepatic encephalopathy compared standard of care with pretreatment with broad-spectrum antibiotics followed by fecal microbiota transplant from a single donor with an "optimal" microbiota found some benefit. The authors found decreased incidence of further hepatic encephalopathy, improved cognition, and increased diversity and beneficial taxa.[29]

Just as with probiotics, more data are needed before fecal microbiota transplants can be recommended as a potential therapy for even refractory recurrent hepatic encephalopathy.

Zinc

Zinc is an essential trace element vital for the activity of urea cycle enzymes as well as glutamine synthetase in muscle cells. For this reason, zinc deficiency, noted to be common among patients with cirrhosis, has been postulated to be directly linked to an increase in serum ammonia levels.[30] However, although this mechanistic link seems clear, the data for zinc supplementation to treat or prevent hepatic encephalopathy remain less clear. Older studies demonstrating conflicting results for the benefit of zinc supplementation have more recently been criticized because many of these studies also involved protein restriction, which as noted above is now thought to be detrimental in the prevention of hepatic encephalopathy, and newer studies are sparse. Takuma and colleagues' 2010 study of 79 patients with cirrhosis and hepatic encephalopathy randomized patients to either zinc in addition to standard therapy, defined as protein-restriction with branched-chain amino acids and lactulose, or standard therapy alone. They found that in multivariate analysis, zinc supplementation improved physical component scales but not mental component scales.[31] A systematic review of 4 trials with 233 patients, including the previously mentioned trial by Takuma and colleagues, found that zinc supplementation was not associated with encephalopathy recurrence, mortality, liver-related morbidity, or quality of life.[32]

ʟ-Ornithine-ʟ-Aspartate

ʟ-ornithine-ʟ-aspartate (LOLA) is thought to lower serum ammonia levels via the activation of carbamyl phosphate synthetase, which converts ammonia to urea, as well as glutamine synthetase, which metabolizes ammonia to glutamine. A 2015 systemic review of 28 RCTs looking available therapies for hepatic encephalopathy, LOLA improved clinical efficacy when compared with no intervention more so than any other intervention (OR, 3.71; CI, 1.98–6.98). However, no statistically significant difference was seen when comparing LOLA directly to other standard therapies including lactulose and rifaximin.[33] A 2019 meta-analysis of 10 RCTs with 919 patients showed a benefit for both low-grade and high-grade hepatic encephalopathies, including improvement in metal state grade by West Haven, psychometric testing, and fasting blood ammonia. When compared with lactulose, rifaximin, probiotics, and branched-chain amino acids, LOLA was found to be equally efficacious, with a possible trend toward superiority.[34] More recently, a 2020 phase 2b trial of a related ammonia scavenger, ornithine phenylacetate, found no difference in median time to improvement when compared with placebo.[35] However, well-designed, large RCTs remain lacking, and despite being used in other countries, LOLA remains inaccessible in the United States.

CLINICS CARE POINTS

- Patients with overt hepatic encephalopathy have been shown to benefit from a restrictive number of pharmacologic therapies. The most commonly used and evidence-based therapies include nonabsorbable disaccharides (e.g. lactulose) and the minimally absorbed oral antibiotic rifaximin.

- The 2014 HELP trial demonstrated promising results for the use of polyethylene glycol in hepatic encephalopathy. Similarly, the 2023 HEAL study demonstrated promising results for the use of albumin. Both of these medications are readily available across healthcare facilities, however more robust data is needed before their use can be recommended as a first line agent alongside lactulose and rifaximin.

• Studies on branched-chain amino acids, probiotics, zinc supplementation, and L-ornithine-L-aspartate (LOLA) have all demonstrated mixed results, and so their use for the treatment of hepatic encephalopathy must be considered on a case-by-case basis.

DISCLOSURE

No disclosures related to the article.

REFERENCES

1. Baertl JM, Sancetta SM, Gabuzda GJ. Relation of acute potassium depletion to renal ammonium metabolism in patients with cirrhosis. The Journal of clinical investigation 1963;42(5):696–706.
2. Maiwall R, Kumar S, Sharma MK, et al. Prevalence and prognostic significance of hyperkalemia in hospitalized patients with cirrhosis. J Gastroenterol Hepatol 2016;31(5):988–94.
3. Ullah H, Shabana H, Rady MA, et al. Hypokalemia as a responsible factor related with the severity of hepatic encephalopathy: a wide multi-nation cross-sectional study. Annals of Medicine and Surgery 2023;10–97.
4. Elkington SG. Lactulose. Gut 1970;11(12):1043.
5. Elkington SG, Floch MH, Conn HO. Lactulose in the treatment of chronic portal-systemic encephalopathy: a double-blind clinical trial. N Engl J Med 1969;281(8):408–12.
6. Gluud LL, Vilstrup H, Morgan MY. Non-absorbable disaccharides versus placebo/no intervention and lactulose versus lactitol for the prevention and treatment of hepatic encephalopathy in people with cirrhosis. Cochrane Database Syst Rev 2016;(4).
7. Dhiman RK, Thumburu KK, Verma N, et al. Comparative efficacy of treatment options for minimal hepatic encephalopathy: a systematic review and network meta-analysis. Clin Gastroenterol Hepatol 2020;18(4):800–12.
8. Sharma BC, Sharma P, Lunia MK, et al. A randomized, double-blind, controlled trial comparing rifaximin plus lactulose with lactulose alone in treatment of overt hepatic encephalopathy. Official journal of the American College of Gastroenterology| ACG 2013;108(9):1458–63.
9. Huang E, Esrailian E, Spiegel BM. The cost-effectiveness and budget impact of competing therapies in hepatic encephalopathy–a decision analysis. Alimentary pharmacology & therapeutics 2007;26(8):1147–61.
10. Agrawal A, Sharma BC, Sharma P, et al. Secondary prophylaxis of hepatic encephalopathy in cirrhosis: an open-label, randomized controlled trial of lactulose, probiotics, and no therapy. Official journal of the American College of Gastroenterology| ACG 2012;107(7):1043–50.
11. Rahimi RS, Singal AG, Cuthbert JA, et al. Lactulose vs polyethylene glycol 3350-electrolyte solution for treatment of overt hepatic encephalopathy: the HELP randomized clinical trial. JAMA Intern Med 2014;174(11):1727–33.
12. Hoilat GJ, Ayas MF, Hoilat JN, et al. Polyethylene glycol versus lactulose in the treatment of hepatic encephalopathy: a systematic review and meta-analysis. BMJ Open Gastroenterology 2021;8(1):e000648.

13. Orlandi F, Freddara U, Candelaresi MT, et al. Comparison between neomycin and lactulose in 173 patients with hepatic encephalopathy: a randomized clinical study. Dig Dis Sci 1981;26:498–506.
14. Strauss E, Tramote R, Silva EP, et al. Double-blind randomized clinical trial comparing neomycin and placebo in the treatment of exogenous hepatic encephalopathy. Hepato-Gastroenterology 1992;39(6):542–5.
15. Berk DP, Chalmers T. Deafness complicating antibiotic therapy of hepatic encephalopathy. Ann Intern Med 1970;73(3):393–6.
16. Bajaj JS. Potential mechanisms of action of rifaximin in the management of hepatic encephalopathy and other complications of cirrhosis. Alimentary pharmacology & therapeutics 2016;43:11–26.
17. Mas A, Rodés J, Sunyer L, et al. Comparison of rifaximin and lactitol in the treatment of acute hepatic encephalopathy: results of a randomized, double-blind, double-dummy, controlled clinical trial. Journal of hepatology 2003;38(1):51–8.
18. Kimer N, et al. Systematic review with meta-analysis: the effects of rifaximin in hepatic encephalopathy. Alimentary pharmacology & therapeutics 2014;40(2): 123–32.
19. Bass NM, et al. Rifaximin treatment in hepatic encephalopathy. N Engl J Med 2010;362(12):1071–81.
20. Bajaj JS, Hassanein TI, Pyrsopoulos NT, et al. Dosing of rifaximin soluble solid dispersion tablets in adults with cirrhosis: 2 randomized, placebo-controlled trials. Clin Gastroenterol Hepatol 2023;21(3):723–31.
21. Simón-Talero M, García-Martínez R, Torrens M, et al. Effects of intravenous albumin in patients with cirrhosis and episodic hepatic encephalopathy: a randomized double-blind study. J Hepatol 2013;59(6):1184–92.
22. Teh KB, Loo JH, Tam YC, et al. Efficacy and safety of albumin infusion for overt hepatic encephalopathy: a systematic review and meta-analysis. Dig Liver Dis 2021;53(7):817–23.
23. Fagan A, Gavis EA, Gallagher ML, et al. A double-blind randomized placebo-controlled trial of albumin in outpatients with hepatic encephalopathy: HEAL study. J Hepatol 2023;78(2):312–21.
24. Iqbal U, Jadeja RN, Khara HS, et al. A comprehensive review evaluating the impact of protein source (vegetarian vs. meat based) in hepatic encephalopathy. Nutrients 2021;13(2):370.
25. Gluud LL, Dam G, Les I, et al. Branched-chain amino acids for people with hepatic encephalopathy. Cochrane Database Syst Rev 2015;(9).
26. Bajaj JS, Saeian K, Christensen KM, et al. Probiotic yogurt for the treatment of minimal hepatic encephalopathy. Official journal of the American College of Gastroenterology| ACG 2008;103(7):1707–15.
27. Dalal R, McGee RG, Riordan SM, et al. Probiotics for people with hepatic encephalopathy. Cochrane Database Syst Rev 2017;(2).
28. Lunia MK, Sharma BC, Sharma P, et al. Probiotics prevent hepatic encephalopathy in patients with cirrhosis: a randomized controlled trial. Clin Gastroenterol Hepatol 2014;12(6):1003–8.
29. Bajaj JS, Kassam Z, Fagan A, et al. Fecal microbiota transplant from a rational stool donor improves hepatic encephalopathy: a randomized clinical trial. Hepatology 2017;66(6):1727–38.
30. Van Der Rijt CC, Schalm SW, Schat H, et al. Overt hepatic encephalopathy precipitated by zinc deficiency. Gastroenterology 1991;100(4):1114–8.
31. Takuma Y, Nouso K, Makino Y, et al. Clinical trial: oral zinc in hepatic encephalopathy. Alimentary pharmacology & therapeutics 2010;32(9):1080–90.

32. Chavez-Tapia NC, Cesar-Arce A, Barrientos-Gutiérrez T, et al. A systematic review and meta-analysis of the use of oral zinc in the treatment of hepatic encephalopathy. Nutr J 2013;12(1):1–6.
33. Zhu GQ, Shi KQ, Huang S, et al. Systematic review with network meta-analysis: the comparative effectiveness and safety of interventions in patients with overt hepatic encephalopathy. Alimentary pharmacology & therapeutics 2015;41(7):624–35.
34. Butterworth RF, McPhail MJ. L-Ornithine L-Aspartate (LOLA) for hepatic encephalopathy in cirrhosis: results of randomized controlled trials and meta-analyses. Drugs 2019;79(Suppl 1):31–7.
35. Rahimi RS, Safadi R, Thabut D, et al. Efficacy and safety of ornithine phenylacetate for treating overt hepatic encephalopathy in a randomized trial. Clin Gastroenterol Hepatol 2021;19(12):2626–35.

Nontraditional Treatment of Hepatic Encephalopathy

Jasleen Singh, MD[a],*, Brittney Ibrahim, BS[b],
Steven-Huy Han, MD[a,b]

KEYWORDS

- Nontraditional treatments • gut microbiome • Probiotics
- Fecal microbiota transplant • Branched chain amino acids • Ammonia
- Albumin dialysis • Liver transplantation

KEY POINTS

- Hyperammonemia is critical to the development of hepatic encephalopathy (HE) but multiple factors contribute to its pathophysiology, including the gut microbiome.
- Traditional treatments of HE such as lactulose and rifaximin target hyperammonemia.
- Nontraditional treatments are broadly classified into gut microbiome modulation, ammonia detoxification, and procedural treatments.
- Many nontraditional treatments such as fecal microbiota transplant, L-ornithine L-aspartate, glycerol phenylbutyrate, and liver support devices are experimental but can be considered in refractory cases.

INTRODUCTION

Hepatic encephalopathy (HE) is defined as brain dysfunction due to liver insufficiency and/or portosystemic shunting ranging from subclinical signs and symptoms to comatose state.[1] It occurs in about 30% to 40% of patients with cirrhosis at some point in their clinical course.[1] HE is classified into 3 types based on clinical presentation: type A is seen in patients with acute liver failure, type B occurs in patients with a portosystemic shunt, and type C refers to HE in patients with cirrhosis with or without a shunt.[2] HE is further divided into overt HE (OHE) and minimal HE (MHE). OHE is defined as clinically evident HE occurring intermittently or persistently with at least 2 episodes during a 6-month period.[1,2] MHE presents with minimal or no clinical signs and symptoms but manifests as abnormalities on psychometric testing.[2] Data show that up to 80% of patients with cirrhosis may have MHE.[3]

---

[a] Department of Medicine, University of California at Los Angeles; Los Angeles, CA, USA;
[b] Department of Surgery, University of California at Los Angeles; Los Angeles, CA, USA
* Corresponding author. Pfleger Liver Institute, UCLA Medical Center, 100 Medical Plaza, Suite 700, Los Angeles, CA 90095.
E-mail address: jassingh@mednet.ucla.edu

Clin Liver Dis 28 (2024) 297–315
https://doi.org/10.1016/j.cld.2024.01.007
1089-3261/24/© 2024 Elsevier Inc. All rights reserved.

Pathophysiology

Altered ammonia (NH_3) clearance leading to a pathogenic hyperammonemic state plays a key role in the development of HE.[4] Ammonia is the end product of protein digestion, amino acid deamination, and urease-producing bacteria.[5] Although the majority of its production takes place in the gut, ammonia is also generated by the brain, muscle, and kidneys.[6] Ammonia is then converted to urea in the liver via the urea cycle and subsequently excreted by the kidneys (75%) and intestine (25%).[5]

In liver failure, ammonia is not adequately cleared by the hepatic urea cycle, thus leading to the accumulation of ammonia in the blood, which crosses the blood–brain barrier.[4] Glutamine synthetase within cerebral astrocytes converts ammonia to glutamine, causing an osmotic effect with astrocyte edema and additional downstream effects including the generation of reactive oxygen species with subsequent cerebral dysfunction.[4,7] Glutamine is also a precursor for the main excitatory and inhibitory neurotransmitters, and thus, its accumulation can alter neurotransmission.[4] **Fig. 1** demonstrates the complexities of HE pathogenesis.

Diagnosis and Management

For OHE, the most commonly used criteria for diagnosis are the West Haven criteria, which are subject to variability between providers.[8] However, diagnosis of MHE relies on objective and reliable tools for diagnosis such as electroencephalogram, continuous reaction time test, inhibitory control test, and computerized test batteries.[9] The Psychometric Hepatic Encephalopathy Score (PHES) has been standardized as

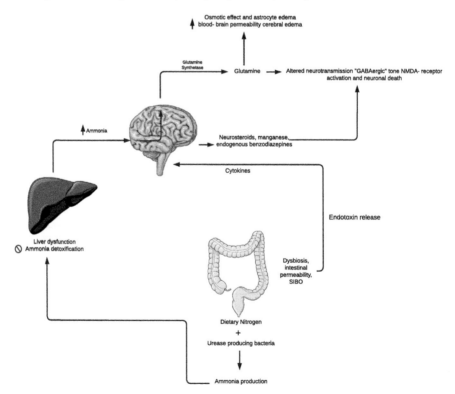

Fig. 1. Pathophysiology of hepatic encephalopathy.

a diagnostic tool in many countries around the world and is the sum score of the 5 subtests: number connection tests A and B, digital symbol test, serial dotting test, and line tracing test.[9]

First-line treatment is the nonabsorbable disaccharides (lactulose and lactitol) that alter ammonia production and metabolism through 4 distinct mechanisms, depicted in **Fig. 2**.[1,2,7,10–12] Lactulose can be administered orally or rectally with the goal of 2 to 3 bowel movements daily.[1,11]

Rifaximin, a nonabsorbable antibiotic, is widely regarded as an adjunctive therapy to lactulose. Studies have shown that combination therapy with lactulose and rifaximin for HE increased clinical efficacy and reduced mortality compared with lactulose alone.[13,14]

GUT-LIVER-BRAIN AXIS

The gut-liver-brain axis is paramount in HE, with multiple gut-related factors affecting cerebral function.[8] Indeed, the known triggers precipitating HE are common gut-related events such as spontaneous bacterial peritonitis (SBP), gastrointestinal bleeding, constipation, and opiate use.[8] Although ammonia production in the gut is critical to the development of HE, liver disease itself alters intestinal function, which may predispose to the development of HE.

Dysbiosis and intestinal permeability are 2 key factors that directly affect progression of liver disease and HE.[7,15,16] Dysbiosis refers to altered bacterial composition in the gastrointestinal tract, leading to an imbalance of beneficial and harmful bacteria. Both dysbiosis and intestinal permeability can result in endotoxemia and activation of inflammatory cytokines, which then increase blood–brain permeability and cerebral edema.[7,17] Small intestinal bacterial overgrowth, another gut-associated condition

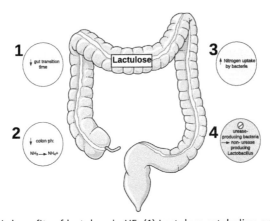

Fig. 2. Therapeutic benefits of lactulose in HE. (1) Lactulose catabolism acidifies the colonic pH, thereby converting ammonia (NH_3) to ammonium (NH_4), which is an impermeable molecule.[7,10,11] (2) Via its laxative effects, lactulose shortens gut transit time, leading to less absorption of ammonia and increase in its excretion.[7,10,11] (3) Lactulose promotes the uptake of nitrogen by bacteria in the colon for protein synthesis.[7,10,11] (4) Lactulose displaces urease-producing bacteria with nonurease producing *Lactobacillus*.[7,10,11] Odeh, M. (2007), Pathogenesis of hepatic encephalopathy: the tumour necrosis factor-α theory. European Journal of Clinical Investigation, 37: 291-304. https://doi.org/10.1111/j.1365-2362.2007. 01778.x.

commonly found in patients with cirrhosis, further alters gut homeostasis by translocation of colonic bacteria into the small intestine, facilitating the release of endotoxins.[18]

Gut Microbiome and Hepatic Encephalopathy

Given the central role the gut plays in ammonia production and metabolism, dysbiosis has also been associated with the development of HE.[19–21] Bajaj and colleagues discovered that *Alcaligenaceae* and *Porphyromonadaceae* were associated with poor cognitive performance, and *Enterobacteriaceae* was associated with worsening inflammation and Model for Endstage Liver Disease (MELD) score in patients with cirrhosis.[19] Bloom and colleagues found a relative decrease in *Anaeromassilibacillus* sp, *Anaerostipes caccae*, *Bacteroides eggerthii*, *Clostridium* sp, *Faecalicatena contorta*, *Holdemania filiformis*, *Neglecta timonensis*, and *Ruminococcus* sp in patients with cirrhosis and OHE.[20]

The gut microbiome also directly impacts brain function with one study demonstrating that pathogenic bacteria were associated with hyperammonemia-associated astrocytic changes and diffuse white matter interstitial edema, which can be seen in HE.[21] These studies support the critical role of the gut microbiome in the progression of HE.

NONTRADITIONAL TREATMENTS OF HEPATIC ENCEPHALOPATHY

Multiple treatment modalities have been developed for a synergistic effect in HE as well as for use in refractory cases. The broad categories of these treatments include gut microbiome modulation, ammonia detoxification, and procedural treatments, as seen in **Fig. 3**. Mechanisms of action of medical therapies are elucidated in **Table 1**.

Gut Microbiome Modulation

Probiotics, prebiotics and synbiotics

Probiotics are defined by the Food and Drug Administration (FDA) and World Health Organization as "live microorganisms which when administered in adequate amounts confer a health benefit to the host."[22] Many popular species include those of the Lactobacillus family, *Bifidobacterium*, nonpathogenic strains of *Escherichia coli*, *Streptococcus salivarius*, *Saccharomyces boulardii*, and VSL#3.[22,23] VSL#3 is the most-studied probiotic in gastrointestinal and liver diseases, consisting of 4 strains of Lactobacillus, 3 strains of *Bifidobacterium*, and 1 strain of *Streptococcus*.[23] Prebiotics are nondigestible food ingredients, such as lactulose, which stimulate the growth of "beneficial" gut bacteria such as *Lactobacillus* and *Bifidobacterium*.[22] Synbiotics represent a combination of prebiotics and probiotics that work in synergy to facilitate the survival of the live microorganisms.[22] The mechanisms by which probiotics alter gut flora and ammonia metabolism are multifactorial. Probiotics may decrease ammonia by (1) decreasing bacterial urease activity, (2) decreasing pH and thus, decreasing absorption of ammonia, (3) decreasing intestinal permeability, and (4) promoting a nutritious environment for the gut epithelium.[24] Probiotics, prebiotics, and synbiotics are a viable treatment target for HE to promote a more favorable gut microbiome that may also modulate systemic inflammation.[25]

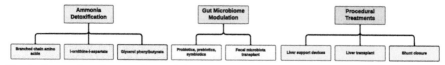

Fig. 3. Categories of nontraditional therapies for treatment of hepatic encephalopathy.

Table 1
Mechanisms of action of nontraditional medical therapies for treatment of hepatic encephalopathy

Therapy	Mechanism of Action
Gut microbiome modulation	
Probiotics, prebiotics, and synbiotics	• ↓ bacterial urease activity and intestinal permeability[24] • ↓ pH → decrease absorption of ammonia[24] • Promote a nutritious environment for the gut epithelium[24]
FMT	• Promotes a more favorable gut environment by reducing urease-producing bacteria[36] • Improves gut integrity → ↓ ammonia absorption into the circulation[36] • ↑ hepatic clearance of ammonia[36]
Ammonia detoxification	
BCAAs	• ↓ the state of malnutrition and protein[43] • Enhances glutamine synthetase activity → ↑ ammonia detoxification[43]
LOLA	• Detoxifies ammonia by promoting conversion to urea and glutamine[47]
GPB	• Promotes nitrogen excretion through formation of PAGN → provides an alternative pathway for nitrogen excess and ammonia[49,50]
Zinc	• Acts as an essential enzymatic cofactor in the urea and glutamine synthetase cycles[53,54]
Sodium benzoate	• Conjugated to hippurate, which contains waste nitrogen → renally excreted[57] • Serves as alternative pathway for ammonia removal[57]

Multiple randomized controlled trials (RCTs) and meta-analyses have been published to examine the effects of probiotics on HE with mixed results, noted in **Table 2**.[26–32] One meta-analysis from 2015 analyzed 14 RCTs with 1152 patients to evaluate the use of probiotics on mortality, improvement in MHE, progression to OHE in patients with MHE, and hospitalizations.[28] The authors found that when compared with placebo or no treatment, probiotics were associated with improvement in MHE (OR: 3.91, 95% CI: 2.25–6.80, $P < .00001$), reduction in hospitalizations (OR: 0.53, 95% CI: 0.33–0.86, $P = .01$), and decreased progression to HE (OR: 0.40, 95% CI: 0.26–0.60, $P < .0001$); however, there was no difference in these outcomes or mortality (OR: 0.69, 95% CI: 0.42–1.14, $P = .15$ and OR: 1.07, 95% CI: 0.47–2.44, $P = .88$, respectively) when compared with lactulose.[28]

Following that meta-analysis, a Cochrane review from 2017 of 21 RCTs with 1420 patients found a high risk of bias in the majority of studies and overall underwhelming results. The authors concluded that while there was little to no difference in mortality when compared with placebo, probiotics may improve recovery from HE and prevent progression to OHE but that the overall quality of evidence was low.[29]

Published in 2018, another meta-analysis of 14 RCTs with 1132 patients demonstrated that probiotics compared with no treatment or placebo were more likely to lower time on the number connection test (mean difference = −30.25, 95% CI: −49.85 to −10.66), improve MHE (OR = 0.18, 95% CI: 0.07–0.47), and prevent progression to OHE (OR = 0.22, 95% CI: 0.07–0.6) at 4 weeks.[30] Compared with lactulose, probiotics tended to reduce serum ammonia levels (mean difference = −0.33 µmol/L, 95% CI: −5.39–4.74), improve MHE (OR = 0.93, 95% CI: 0.45–1.91) and prevent the

Table 2
Studies of probiotics, prebiotics, and synbiotics in patients with hepatic encephalopathy

Authors	# Trials/Patients	Intervention	Outcomes	Results Compared to NT/Placebo	Results Compared with Lactulose
Saab S, et al,[28] 2016	14/1152	Probiotics vs lactulose, NT/placebo	Mortality, improvement in MHE, hospitalizations, and progression to OHE	• ↓ MHE, ↓ hospitalization rates, ↓ progression to OHE • No Δ mortality	• No Δ MHE, hospitalizations, progression to OHE • No Δ mortality
Cao Q, et al,[30] 2018	14/1132	Probiotics vs lactulose, NT/placebo	NCT values, improvement in MHE, progression to OHE, and ammonia	• ↓ values NCT, ↓ MHE, ↓ progression to OHE	• ↓ trend in ammonia, ↓ values NCT, ↓ MHE, ↓ OHE • Lactulose more significantly reduced NCT values
Dalal R, et al,[29] 2017	21/1420	Probiotics vs lactulose, NT/placebo	Mortality, no recovery, hospitalizations, quality of life (QOL), and ammonia	• No Δ mortality, ↓ no recovery, ? effect on hospitalizations, may ↑ QOL, ↓ ammonia	• ? effects given low quality of evidence
Xu J, Ma R, Chen LF, Zhao LJ, Chen K, Zhang RB[67]	6/496	Probiotics vs NT/placebo	Development of OHE, mortality, ammonia, and constipation	• ↓ development of OHE but no Δ mortality, ammonia, and constipation	
Zhao LN, et al,[68] 2014	9/-	Probiotics vs NT/placebo	Improvement of MHE, prevention of OHE, ammonia, physical and psychosocial sickness impact profile (SIP), hospitalizations, infections, and unrelated ER visits	• ↓ MHE, prevention of OHE, ↓ ammonia, ↓ physical and psychosocial SIP, ↓ hospitalizations, ↓ infections, ↓ unrelated ER visits	

Study		Intervention	Outcomes	Results	
Holte K, et al,[69] 2012	7/393	Probiotics or synbiotics vs lactulose, and NT/placebo	Improvement in HE, ammonia, and psychometric tests	• ↓ HE, ↓ arterial ammonia, no Δ psychometric tests	• ↓ HE, ↓ arterial ammonia, no Δ psychometric tests
Shukla S, et al,[70] 2011	9/349	Prebiotics, probiotics, and synbiotics	Improvement of MHE	• ↓ risk of no improvement of MHE • 5 studies with lactulose ↓ risk of no improvement of MHE	
McGee RG, et al,[71] 2011	7/550	Probiotics vs lactulose and placebo, NT/placebo	Mortality, lack of recovery, QOL, and ammonia	• No Δ mortality, lack of recovery, QOL	• No Δ lack of recovery, ammonia
Huang L, et al,[72] 2022	17/-	Probiotics, lactulose, and placebo	Ammonia, incidence of HE, mortality, and SBP	• ↓ ammonia and HE, no Δ SBP and mortality	• ↓ ammonia, no Δ decreasing incidence of HE

Abbreviations: ER, emergency room; NCT, number connection test.

development of OHE (OR = 0.96, 95% CI: 0.17–5.44) at 4 weeks.[30] Again, however, the studies included were of low overall quality.

While probiotics have a theoretic benefit in the treatment of HE and despite the sheer number of studies that have been conducted to examine this, most of the studies are of low quality and thus, probiotics are not routinely recommended for the treatment or prevent of HE.

Fecal microbiota transplant

Fecal microbiota transplant (FMT) is indicated for the treatment of certain gut diseases such as *Clostridium difficile* and ulcerative colitis due to the dysfunctional gut microbiome that is central to these illnesses.[33–35] As the pathogenesis of HE is similarly associated with dysbiosis, FMT could be a potential treatment for patients with HE. FMT theoretically promotes a more favorable gut environment by (1) reducing urease-producing bacteria, (2) improving gut integrity leading to reduced ammonia absorption into the circulation, and (3) increasing hepatic clearance of ammonia.[36] FMT is administered to the colon through the upper gastrointestinal tract via nasoduodenal tube or capsule or directly into the colon with colonoscopy or enema.[37]

The first RCT to study FMT in HE was by Bajaj and colleagues in 2017. In this study, 20 patients with at least 2 episodes of OHE were randomized 1:1 to FMT enema with the use of pre-FMT antibiotics or standard of care (SOC).[38] A single donor for FMT was used with high abundance of *Lachnospiraceae* and *Ruminococcaceae*, which are considered beneficial autochthonous taxa.[38] Patients in the FMT group had an improvement in the PHES score ($P = .003$) and EncephalApp Stroop ($P = .01$) from baseline values as compared with the SOC arm that demonstrated no improvement with a follow-up of 150 days postrandomization.[38] The authors noted an increase in abundance of *Lachnospiraceae* and *Ruminococcaceae* compared with postantibiotics microbiome.[38] A long-term analysis was also performed to evaluate outcomes during 12 months.[39] In the FMT arm compared with the SOC arm at 12 months, there were fewer hospitalizations ($P = .05$), no HE events (compared with 8 HE events in the SOC arm, $P = .03$) and sustained improvement in cognitive function.[39]

Although enemas are one method of FMT delivery, other mechanisms such as an FMT capsule, which may be more palatable for patients, are available. A phase 1, placebo-controlled trial was performed to evaluate its safety and efficacy in HE.[40] Twenty patients were randomized 1:1 to FMT capsule or placebo with a primary outcome of safety and tolerability.[40] FMT capsule met the primary outcome. Additionally, patients post-FMT capsule demonstrated increased diversity of duodenal flora ($P = .01$) with a higher abundance of Ruminococcaceae and Bifidobacteriaceae and lower abundance of Streptococcaceae and Veillonellaceae.[40] Patients given FMT capsule exhibited improved performance with EncephalApp ($P = .02$) but no improvement in PHES.[40]

A subsequent open-label trial in 2022 studied FMT capsule in 10 patients with cirrhosis and OHE.[41] The authors aimed to study multiple donors and evaluate recipient factors related to the success of FMT capsule in patients with OHE.[41] Mean improvement of PHES was 3.1 points in patients after receiving 5 doses of FMT capsules given over 3 weeks.[41] FMT capsule was efficacious, with only one patient (10%) experiencing OHE after 6 months of follow-up.[41] One key finding was that outcomes varied depending on donor FMT. One donor in particular led to a worse outcome for the recipient. This donor was found to have lower short chain fatty acid levels and alterations in bile acids, which are known to protect gut integrity.[41] Although the authors did not find wholesale remodeling of the gut microbiome, FMT may promote modulation of gut permeability, mitigation of immune response, and improved sensitivity to antibiotics such as rifaximin to exert its benefit in HE.[41]

Table 3
Studies of fecal microbiota transplant in patients with hepatic encephalopathy

Study	Type of Study	# Of Patients	Intervention	Outcomes	Results
Bajaj et al,[38] 2017	Open-label RCT, 1:1 randomization	20	FMT enema (single donor, use of pretreatment antibiotics) vs SOC with up to 5-mo follow-up	• Primary: SAEs, composite end point of death, hospitalizations, ER visits, and transmissible infections • Secondary: changes in cognitive function at day 20, cirrhosis severity (MELD score, albumin), changes in liver function and WBC count, development of all AEs, and changes in microbiota composition and function	• 20% SAEs in FMT arm compared with 80% SAEs in SOC arm (mostly liver-related) • No HE episodes at 150 d in FMT arm compared with 6 HE episodes in SOC arm (P = .03) • Improvement in PHES and EncephalApp Stroop (P = .01) compared with baseline values and no improvement in SOC arm • Changes in microbiota composition in FMT arm
Bajaj et al,[39] 2019	Long-term analysis of previous trial over more than 12 mo				• Fewer hospitalizations in FMT arm (P = .05) • No HE events (compared with 8 in the SOC arm) (P = .03) • Sustained improvement in cognitive function

(continued on next page)

Table 3
(continued)

Study	Type of Study	# Of Patients	Intervention	Outcomes	Results
Bajaj et al,[40] 2019	Placebo-controlled, phase 1 RCT, 1:1 randomization	20	FMT capsule from a single donor vs placebo capsules	Primary: SAEs, safety and tolerability • Secondary: AEs other than hospitalization/ER visits, changes in mucosal and stool microbiota, changes in PHES and EncephalApp, serum LBP, changes in duodenal mucosal cytokines, barrier proteins, and AMPs	• Met primary outcome of safety and tolerability • Not powered for efficacy – trended toward fewer hospitalizations but not HE • Improvement in EncephalApp performance ($P = .02$) in FMT group but not PHES • Increased duodenal mucosal diversity, changes in cytokines and barrier proteins, and reduced LBP levels post-FMT
Bloom et al,[41] 2022	Open-label single-arm study	10	FMT capsules from multiple donors	Safety, change in PHES, change in EncephalApp Stroop Test, stool analysis, and inflammatory biomarkers	• 3 SAEs – 1 before trial, 1 ESBL *E coli* bacteremia, 1 decompensation after missing lactulose • PHES improved 4 wk after fifth dose of FMT (+3.1, $P = .02$) • No change in Stroop but trended toward improvement 4 wk after fifth dose of FMT (19.1 s improved, $P = .05$)

- 7 patients responded to FMT with improved PHES and no OHE at 6 mo
- No change in inflammatory markers
- No significant remodeling of microbiome
- Outcomes varied by donor

Abbreviations: AMP, adenosine monophosphate.

Table 3 includes the available trials of FMT and HE. Future larger-scale trials are needed before FMT can be considered a viable therapeutic option for HE.

Ammonia Detoxification

Branched chain amino acids

Branched chain amino acids (BCAAs), including valine, leucine, and isoleucine, as a source of protein and promotor of muscle detoxification of ammonia have been studied as potential treatment in HE.[42] Although the exact mechanism of BCAAs in HE is unknown, the suggested mechanisms by which BCAAs contribute to ammonia detoxification occur via increase in skeletal muscle mass.[43] BCAAs may reduce the state of malnutrition and protein breakdown that occurs in decompensated liver disease and HE.[43] This increase in muscle mass also enhances glutamine synthetase activity, which increases ammonia detoxification.[43]

A meta-analysis in 2017 evaluated 16 RCTs with 827 patients to understand the impact of oral and intravenous BCAAs on OHE and MHE.[43] The authors found a beneficial effect of BCAAs on HE (RR: 0.73, 95% CI: 0.61–0.88), and this benefit persisted even when including only the trials with a low risk of bias (RR: 0.71, 95% CI: 0.52–0.96). However, the only high-quality RCT published in 2011 did not show that BCAAs decreased the recurrence of HE.[2,44] Therefore, there are insufficient data at present to recommend BCAAs in the treatment of HE, and higher quality studies are needed to examine their effects.

L-ornithine L-aspartate

Although the data to use BCAAs in HE are lacking, the data for L-ornithine L-aspartate (LOLA) are more robust. LOLA is a mixture of 2 amino acids and is thought to stimulate urea synthesis and ammonia conversion to glutamine.[45,46] By providing substrates and activating the urea cycle, LOLA is thought to detoxify ammonia by promoting conversion to urea and glutamine.[47] Multiple meta-analyses and systematic reviews have been published on LOLA and HE.[45]

A Cochrane review published in 2018 included the results of 29 RCTs (of which only 5 trials were considered to be low risk of bias) and 1891 patients with the majority of studies looking at the treatment of HE.[48] When analyzing all trials, LOLA compared with placebo or no intervention did have a beneficial effect on mortality (RR: 0.42, 95% CI: 0.24–0.72; I^2 = 0%) and HE (RR: 0.70, 95% CI: 0.59–0.83; 22 trials; 1375 participants; I^2 = 62%). However, this effect was not seen when considering only trials with low risk of bias.[48] LOLA was also compared with probiotics, lactulose, and rifaximin. In these studies, LOLA had no significant effect when compared with lactulose and rifaximin on mortality, HE, or adverse events.[48]

A study from 2022 evaluated 140 patients with grade III-IV HE receiving lactulose and rifaximin randomized to 5 days of treatment with LOLA versus placebo.[46] Patients receiving LOLA had a higher rate of resolution or improvement of HE (88.57% vs 68.57%, P < .001), shorter time to recovery from HE (2.70 ± 0.46 days vs 3.00 ± 0.87 days; P = .03), and lower 28-day mortality (16.4% vs 41.8%, P = .001).

The results of this recent RCT may pave the way for future studies but, at present, LOLA is not routinely used for the treatment of HE.

Glycerol phenylbutyrate

Glycerol phenylbutyrate (GPB) is a prodrug of sodium phenylbutyrate and consists of 3 molecules of phenylbutyric acid (PBA).[49,50] GPB promotes nitrogen excretion through the formation of urinary phenylacetyl glutamine (PAGN), thus providing an alternative pathway for nitrogen excess and ammonia.[49,50] It has been approved for the use of hyperammonemia in urea cycle disorders and thus warrants study in patients with cirrhosis and HE.[50]

A 4-week open-label pilot study in 2013 showed GPB 6 mL bid lowered fasting venous ammonia levels in cirrhotic patients with HE.[51] A follow-up study was a double-blind multicenter RCT in 2014, in which 178 patients with cirrhosis and HE were randomized to GPB 6 mL bid or placebo.[50] Dropout rate was high (63.6% patients in the GPB group and 31.3% in the placebo group).[50] In the intention-to-treat analysis, there was a lower proportion of patients in the GPB arm who experienced an HE event as compared with placebo (21% vs 36%, $P = .02$).[50] Fasting ammonia level was significantly lower in the GPB arm versus placebo ($P = .04$).[50] However, there was no significant difference in HE hospitalizations. Limitations of this study included a high rate of dropout, nonuniform use of rifaximin (only United States patients used rifaximin), and many adverse effects (AEs) reported.[50]

Another study evaluated the use of sodium phenylbutyrate (SPB) in patients with cirrhosis and HE in the intensive care unit. This study found significantly lower levels of ammonia and more neurologic improvement in patients treated with SPB compared with controls (83% vs 50%, $P = .0339$).[52]

Although this medication has been approved for the use of hyperammonemia in urea cycle disorders, there are not enough data to support its routine use in HE.

Zinc

Zinc has been studied for the treatment of HE, although data are conflicting from multiple studies. Zinc is a key enzymatic cofactor in the urea and glutamine synthetase cycles, necessary for the activity of enzymes such as ornithine transcarbamylase and glutamate dehydrogenase.[53,54] In chronic liver disease, there may be zinc deficiency, which decreases the activity of the aforementioned enzymes, leading to an accumulation of ammonia.[55] This highlights the theoretic benefit of zinc as a potential therapy for HE. A meta-analysis published in 2013, based on 4 RCTs studying zinc compared with placebo/no intervention, found only an improvement in the number connection test but failed to demonstrate a statistically significant difference in HE recurrence.[56] Based on the available data, American Association for the Study of Liver Diseases (AASLD) and European Association for the Study of the Liver (EASL) guidelines do not recommend zinc for the treatment of HE.[1,2]

Sodium benzoate

Sodium benzoate is commonly used as a food and beverage preservative and although not FDA-approved, it has been used to treat HE in hyperammonemic states, such as urea cycle disorders.[57] Sodium benzoate is conjugated to hippurate, which contains waste nitrogen that is then renally excreted.[57] One of the first studies to evaluate efficacy of sodium benzoate was published in 1992, randomizing 74 patients with cirrhosis or surgical portosystemic shunts with HE for less than 7 days to sodium benzoate or lactulose.[58] The authors found that 30 patients (80%) receiving sodium benzoate and 29 patients (81%) receiving lactulose recovered ($P > .1$), proving sodium benzoate to be an alternative to the comparatively more expensive lactulose at the time.[58] Another study published in 2020 evaluated sodium benzoate in the pediatric patient population who had decompensated liver disease and hyperammonemia. Patients were randomized to standard therapy and sodium benzoate or standard therapy and placebo, with standard therapy indicating lactulose and rifaximin use. They found that ammonia levels decreased on days 1 and 2 but not subsequently, and there was no significant difference in resolution of HE between the sodium benzoate group compared with placebo (57.1% vs 50%, $P = 1$). Sodium benzoate did not have an impact on other outcomes such as hospital stay, 28-day transplant-free survival, or 90-day transplant-free survival.[59] An additional consideration is the sodium content in sodium benzoate, and it may not be ideal for patients with ascites or edema.[57] In conclusion, sodium benzoate may be a relatively safe and inexpensive addition to standard therapies for HE but more data are needed to make a universal recommendation.

Procedural Treatments

Liver support devices

Artificial liver support systems have been studied in both acute liver failure and acute on chronic liver failure (ACLF), with the molecular adsorbent recirculating system (MARS) being the most studied.[60] The MARS system uses an albumin-enriched dialysate to remove albumin-bound toxins and requires a dialysis machine to function.[61]

A study from 2007 randomized 70 patients in 8 tertiary care centers with HE grade 3 or 4 to extracorporeal albumin dialysis (ECAD) plus standard medical therapy (SMT) or SMT alone.[62] Results showed improvement of HE was higher in the ECAD group versus SMT (34% vs 18.9%, $P = .044$).[62]

Several years later, Bañares and colleagues randomized 189 patients with ACLF to MARS versus SMT and found more improvement of HE from grade 2 to 4 to grade 0 to 1 in the MARS arm, although this was not statistically significant (62.5% vs 38.2%, $P = .07$).[63] Although MARS had an acceptable safety profile, it had no overall impact on survival.[63]

Liver support devices are a feasible option in patients with refractory HE but may not be widely available for use. Per EASL guidelines, albumin dialysis may be considered in HE although there is an uncertain impact on prognosis.[2]

Liver transplantation

Liver transplantation (LT) is generally considered curative for HE in cirrhosis, although it is not necessarily an indication for LT. However, patients with cirrhosis who experience a first episode of OHE have a shorter transplant-free survival; therefore, it is recommended these patients should be referred to a transplant center for evaluation.[64]

In addition to LT considerations, patients with medically refractory HE should be evaluated for the presence of spontaneous portosystemic shunts. A retrospective study of 20 patients with refractory HE from portosytemic shunts at a tertiary center who underwent shunt embolization resulted in immediate improvement in all patients. Most patients experienced durable improvement without HE recurrence after embolization (92%) at 1 year.[65] There are multiple techniques for shunt closure that can be performed by interventional radiology with an acceptable risk profile.[66]

SUMMARY

Abnormalities in ammonia production and metabolism constitute the key factors in the development of HE. Traditional treatments have targeted the hyperammonemic state. However, the etiologies of HE are multifactorial and thus present a myriad of possible treatment targets. The gut microbiome, for example, may be considered a driver in the progression of cognitive dysfunction in cirrhosis, and nontraditional treatments such as probiotics and FMT may be viable alternative therapies for HE. Other nontraditional treatments targeted at the urea cycle or protein synthesis, such as GPB or amino acids, may be considered in refractory cases but are not supported by available data. Further investigation with high-quality studies is warranted to determine the role of gut microbiome modulation and ammonia detoxification in the clinical treatment and resolution of HE. Liver support devices such as MARS offer an alternative to refractory HE cases but are not widely available and may have significant costs associated. Finally, although LT is not warranted in all cases of HE, it remains the definitive treatment for HE in cirrhosis.

CLINICS CARE POINTS

- HE, as a complication of liver disease, is the result of abnormalities in the gut, liver, and brain, with hyperammonemia playing a critical role
- In pathologic states such as cirrhosis and HE, the gut microbiome is altered, leading to a state of imbalance between beneficial and harmful taxa and intestinal permeability
- Treatments for HE such as probiotics and FMT target the gut microbiome and have shown promising results but more high-quality studies are warranted
- Other treatments such as BCAAs, L-ornithine L-aspartate and glycerol phenylbutyrate have been studied as a means of addressing hyperammonemia in HE but are not routinely used in practice
- LT is ultimately considered the curative option for HE

DISCLOSURE

Financial support: None. Conflicts of interest: None.

REFERENCES

1. American Association for the Study of Liver Diseases. European Association for the Study of the Liver. Hepatic encephalopathy in chronic liver disease: 2014 practice guideline by the European Association for the Study of the Liver and the American Association for the Study of Liver Diseases. J Hepatol 2014; 61(3):642–59.
2. European Association for. the Study of the Liver. Electronic address: easloffice@easloffice.eu; European Association for the Study of the Liver. EASL Clinical Practice Guidelines on the management of hepatic encephalopathy. J Hepatol 2022;77(3):807–24.
3. Butterworth RF. Hepatic Encephalopathy in cirrhosis: Pathology and pathophysiology. Drugs 2019 Feb;79(Suppl 1):17–21.
4. Tranah TH, Paolino A, Shawcross DL. Pathophysiological mechanisms of hepatic encephalopathy. Clin Liver Dis 2015;5(3):59–63.
5. Rocco A, Sgamato C, Compare D, et al. Gut Microbes and hepatic encephalopathy: From the old Concepts to new perspectives. Front Cell Dev Biol 2021;9: 748253.
6. Rose CF, Amodio P, Bajaj JS, et al. Hepatic encephalopathy: Novel insights into classification, pathophysiology and therapy. J Hepatol 2020;73(6):1526–47.
7. Hoilat GJ, Suhail FK, Adhami T, et al. Evidence-based approach to management of hepatic encephalopathy in adults. World J Hepatol 2022;14(4):670–81.
8. Bajaj JS. The role of microbiota in hepatic encephalopathy. Gut Microb 2014;5(3): 397–403.

9. Weissenborn K. Diagnosis of minimal hepatic encephalopathy. J Clin Exp Hepatol 2015;5(Suppl 1):S54–9.
10. Wijdicks EF. Hepatic encephalopathy. N Engl J Med 2016;375(17):1660–70.
11. Elwir S, Rahimi RS. Hepatic encephalopathy: an Update on the Pathophysiology and therapeutic options. J Clin Transl Hepatol 2017;5(2):142–51.
12. Mangini C, Montagnese S. New Therapies of liver diseases: hepatic encephalopathy. J Clin Med 2021;10(18):4050.
13. Bass NM, Mullen KD, Sanyal A, et al. Rifaximin treatment in hepatic encephalopathy. N Engl J Med 2010;362(12):1071–81.
14. Wang Z, Chu P, Wang W. Combination of rifaximin and lactulose improves clinical efficacy and mortality in patients with hepatic encephalopathy. Drug Des Devel Ther 2018;13:1–11.
15. Chen Y, Yang F, Lu H, et al. Characterization of fecal microbial communities in patients with liver cirrhosis. Hepatology 2011;54(2):562–72.
16. Bajaj JS, Heuman DM, Hylemon PB, et al. Altered profile of human gut microbiome is associated with cirrhosis and its complications. J Hepatol 2014;60(5):940–7.
17. Tapper EB, Jiang ZG, Patwardhan VR. Refining the ammonia hypothesis: a physiology-driven approach to the treatment of hepatic encephalopathy. Mayo Clin Proc 2015;90(5):646–58.
18. Fukui H. Gut Microbiota and host Reaction in liver diseases. Microorganisms 2015;3(4):759–91.
19. Bajaj JS, Ridlon JM, Hylemon PB, et al. Linkage of gut microbiome with cognition in hepatic encephalopathy. Am J Physiol Gastrointest Liver Physiol 2012;302(1):G168–75.
20. Bloom PP, Luévano JM Jr, Miller KJ, et al. Deep stool microbiome analysis in cirrhosis reveals an association between short-chain fatty acids and hepatic encephalopathy. Ann Hepatol 2021;25:100333.
21. Ahluwalia V, Betrapally NS, Hylemon PB, et al. Impaired gut-liver-brain Axis in Patients with cirrhosis. Sci Rep 2016;6:26800.
22. Pandey KR, Naik SR, Vakil BV. Probiotics, prebiotics and synbiotics- a review. J Food Sci Technol 2015;52(12):7577–87.
23. Cheng FS, Pan D, Chang B, et al. Probiotic mixture VSL#3: An overview of basic and clinical studies in chronic diseases. World J Clin Cases 2020;8(8):1361–84.
24. Poh Z, Chang PE. A current review of the diagnostic and treatment strategies of hepatic encephalopathy. Int J Hepatol 2012;2012:480309.
25. Yadav MK, Kumari I, Singh B, et al. Probiotics, prebiotics and synbiotics: Safe options for next-generation therapeutics. Appl Microbiol Biotechnol 2022 Jan;106(2):505–21.
26. Lunia MK, Sharma BC, Sharma P, et al. Probiotics prevent hepatic encephalopathy in patients with cirrhosis: a randomized controlled trial. Clin Gastroenterol Hepatol 2014 Jun;12(6):1003–8.e1.
27. Bajaj JS, Saeian K, Christensen KM, et al. Probiotic yogurt for the treatment of minimal hepatic encephalopathy. Am J Gastroenterol 2008;103(7):1707–15.
28. Saab S, Suraweera D, Au J, et al. Probiotics are helpful in hepatic encephalopathy: a meta-analysis of randomized trials. Liver Int 2016;36(7):986–93.
29. Dalal R, McGee RG, Riordan SM, et al. Probiotics for people with hepatic encephalopathy. Cochrane Database Syst Rev 2017;2(2):CD008716.
30. Cao Q, Yu CB, Yang SG, et al. Effect of probiotic treatment on cirrhotic patients with minimal hepatic encephalopathy: a meta-analysis. Hepatobiliary Pancreat Dis Int 2018;17(1):9–16.

31. Dhiman RK, Thumburu KK, Verma N, et al. Comparative Efficacy of treatment Options for minimal hepatic encephalopathy: a systematic Review and network meta-analysis. Clin Gastroenterol Hepatol 2020;18(4):800–12.e25.
32. Liu Q, Duan ZP, Ha DK, et al. Synbiotic modulation of gut flora: effect on minimal hepatic encephalopathy in patients with cirrhosis. Hepatology 2004;39(5): 1441–9.
33. Hui W, Li T, Liu W, et al. Fecal microbiota transplantation for treatment of recurrent C. difficile infection: An updated randomized controlled trial meta-analysis. PLoS One 2019;14(1):e0210016.
34. Ishikawa D, Zhang X, Nomura K, et al. A randomized placebo-controlled Trial of combination therapy with post-triple-antibiotic-therapy fecal microbiota Transplantation and Alginate for ulcerative colitis: protocol. Front Med 2022;9:779205.
35. Rossen NG, Fuentes S, van der Spek MJ, et al. Findings From a randomized controlled Trial of fecal Transplantation for patients with ulcerative colitis. Gastroenterology 2015 Jul;149(1):110–8.e4.
36. Madsen M, Kimer N, Bendtsen F, et al. Fecal microbiota transplantation in hepatic encephalopathy: a systematic review. Scand J Gastroenterol 2021;56(5):560–9. Epub 2021 Apr 10. PMID: 33840331.
37. Kim KO, Gluck M. Fecal microbiota transplantation: an Update on clinical practice. Clin Endosc 2019;52(2):137–43.
38. Bajaj JS, Kassam Z, Fagan A, et al. Fecal microbiota transplant from a rational stool donor improves hepatic encephalopathy: a randomized clinical trial. Hepatology 2017;66(6):1727–38.
39. Bajaj JS, Fagan A, Gavis EA, et al. Long-term Outcomes of fecal microbiota Transplantation in patients with cirrhosis. Gastroenterology 2019;156(6): 1921–3.e3.
40. Bajaj JS, Salzman NH, Acharya C, et al. Fecal microbial transplant capsules are Safe in hepatic encephalopathy: a phase 1, randomized, placebo-controlled trial. Hepatology 2019;70(5):1690–703.
41. Bloom PP, Donlan J, Torres Soto M, et al. Fecal microbiota transplant improves cognition in hepatic encephalopathy and its effect varies by donor and recipient. Hepatol Commun 2022;6(8):2079–89.
42. Dam G, Aamann L, Vistrup H, et al. The role of branched chain amino Acids in the treatment of hepatic encephalopathy. J Clin Exp Hepatol 2018;8(4):448–51.
43. Gluud LL, Dam G, Les I, et al. Branched-chain amino acids for people with hepatic encephalopathy. Cochrane Database Syst Rev 2017;5(5):CD001939.
44. Les I, Doval E, García-Martínez R, et al. Effects of branched-chain amino acids supplementation in patients with cirrhosis and a previous episode of hepatic encephalopathy: a randomized study. Am J Gastroenterol 2011;106(6):1081–8.
45. Butterworth RF, McPhail MJW. L-ornithine L-aspartate (LOLA) for hepatic Encephalopathy in cirrhosis: Results of randomized controlled Trials and meta-analyses. Drugs 2019;79(Suppl 1):31–7.
46. Jain A, Sharma BC, Mahajan B, et al. L-ornithine L-aspartate in acute treatment of severe hepatic encephalopathy: a double-blind randomized controlled trial. Hepatology 2022;75(5):1194–203.
47. Kircheis G, Lüth S. Pharmacokinetic and pharmacodynamic Properties of L-ornithine L-aspartate (LOLA) in hepatic encephalopathy. Drugs 2019;79(Suppl 1):23–9.
48. Goh ET, Stokes CS, Sidhu SS, et al. L-ornithine L-aspartate for prevention and treatment of hepatic encephalopathy in people with cirrhosis. Cochrane Database Syst Rev 2018;5. Art. No.: CD012410.

49. McGuire BM, Zupanets IA, Lowe ME, et al. Pharmacology and safety of glycerol phenylbutyrate in healthy adults and adults with cirrhosis. Hepatology 2010 Jun; 51(6):2077–85.

50. Rockey DC, Vierling JM, Mantry P, et al, HALT-HE Study Group. Randomized, double-blind, controlled study of glycerol phenylbutyrate in hepatic encephalopathy. Hepatology 2014;59(3):1073–83.

51. Ghabril M, Zupanets IA, Vierling J, et al. Glycerol Phenylbutyrate in patients with Cirrhosis and episodic hepatic encephalopathy: a pilot Study of Safety and Effect on venous ammonia concentration. Clin Pharmacol Drug Dev 2013;2(3):278–84.

52. Weiss N, Tripon S, Lodey M, et al. Brain-Liver Pitié-Salpêtrière Study Group (BLIPS). Treating hepatic encephalopathy in cirrhotic patients admitted to ICU with sodium phenylbutyrate: a preliminary study. Fundam Clin Pharmacol 2018; 32(2):209–15.

53. Grüngreiff K, Reinhold D, Wedemeyer H. The role of zinc in liver cirrhosis. Ann Hepatol 2016;15(1):7–16.

54. Miwa T, Hanai T, Toshihide M, et al. Zinc deficiency predicts overt hepatic encephalopathy and mortality in liver cirrhosis patients with minimal hepatic encephalopathy. Hepatol Res 2021;51(6):662–73.

55. Katayama K. Zinc and protein metabolism in chronic liver diseases. Nutr Res 2020;74:1–9. Epub 2019 Nov 27. PMID: 31891865.

56. Chavez-Tapia NC, Cesar-Arce A, Barrientos-Gutiérrez T, et al. A systematic review and meta-analysis of the use of oral zinc in the treatment of hepatic encephalopathy. Nutr J 2013;12:74.

57. Misel ML, Gish RG, Patton H, et al. Sodium benzoate for treatment of hepatic encephalopathy. Gastroenterol Hepatol 2013;9(4):219–27. PMID: 24711766; PMCID: PMC3977640.

58. Sushma S, Dasarathy S, Tandon RK, et al. Sodium benzoate in the treatment of acute hepatic encephalopathy: a double-blind randomized trial. Hepatology 1992;16(1):138–44.

59. Snehavardhan P, Lal BB, Sood V, et al. Efficacy and Safety of sodium Benzoate in the Management of Hyperammonemia in decompensated chronic liver Disease of the childhood-A double-blind randomized controlled trial. J Pediatr Gastroenterol Nutr 2020;70(2):165–70. PMID: 31978010.

60. Bañares R, Ibáñez-Samaniego L, Torner JM, et al. Meta-analysis of individual patient data of albumin dialysis in acute-on-chronic liver failure: focus on treatment intensity. Therap Adv Gastroenterol 2019;12. 1756284819879565.

61. Saliba F. The Molecular Adsorbent Recirculating System (MARS) in the intensive care unit: a rescue therapy for patients with hepatic failure. Crit Care 2006; 10(1):118.

62. Hassanein TI, Tofteng F, Brown RS Jr, et al. Randomized controlled study of extracorporeal albumin dialysis for hepatic encephalopathy in advanced cirrhosis. Hepatology 2007;46(6):1853–62.

63. Bañares R, Nevens F, Larsen FS, et al, RELIEF study group. Extracorporeal albumin dialysis with the molecular adsorbent recirculating system in acute-on-chronic liver failure: the RELIEF trial. Hepatology 2013;57(3):1153–62.

64. Bustamante J, Rimola A, Ventura PJ, et al. Prognostic significance of hepatic encephalopathy in patients with cirrhosis. J Hepatol 1999;30(5):890–5.

65. Lynn AM, Singh S, Congly SE, et al. Embolization of portosystemic shunts for treatment of medically refractory hepatic encephalopathy. Liver Transpl 2016; 22(6):723–31.

66. Philips CA, Rajesh S, Augustine P, et al. Portosystemic shunts and refractory hepatic encephalopathy: patient selection and current options. Hepat Med 2019;11: 23–34.
67. Xu J, Ma R, Chen LF, et al. Effects of probiotic therapy on hepatic encephalopathy in patients with liver cirrhosis: an updated meta-analysis of six randomized controlled trials. Hepatobiliary Pancreat Dis Int 2014;13(4):354–60.
68. Zhao LN, Yu T, Lan SY, et al. Probiotics can improve the clinical outcomes of hepatic encephalopathy: An update meta-analysis. Clin Res Hepatol Gastroenterol 2015;39(6):674–82.
69. Holte K, Krag A, Gluud LL. Systematic review and meta-analysis of randomized trials on probiotics for hepatic encephalopathy. Hepatol Res 2012;42(10): 1008–15.
70. Shukla S, Shukla A, Mehboob S, et al. Meta-analysis: the effects of gut flora modulation using prebiotics, probiotics and synbiotics on minimal hepatic encephalopathy. Aliment Pharmacol Ther 2011;33(6):662–71.
71. McGee RG, Bakens A, Wiley K, et al. Probiotics for patients with hepatic encephalopathy. Cochrane Database Syst Rev 2011;(11):CD008716.
72. Huang L, Yu Q, Peng H, et al. Alterations of gut microbiome and effects of probiotic therapy in patients with liver cirrhosis: a systematic review and meta-analysis. Medicine (Baltim) 2022;101(51):e32335.

Interventional Radiology Management of Hepatic Encephalopathy

Edward Wolfgang Lee, MD, PhD[a,b,]*, Justine J. Liang, MD, MS[c],
Griffin P. McNamara, MD[a]

KEYWORDS

- Hepatic encephalopathy • Spontaneous portosystemic shunt
- Transjugular intrahepatic portosystemic shunt • Retrograde transvenous obliteration
- CARTO • TIPS reduction • TIPS occlusion

KEY POINTS

- Hepatic encephalopathy (HE) is a devastating complication of cirrhosis.
- HE in patients with spontaneous portosystemic shunt (spontaneous portosystemic shunt-related HE [SPSS-HE]) is not uncommon.
- SPSS-HE can be effectively treated with shunt embolization (retrograde transvenous obliteration or antegrade transvenous obliteration).
- Posttransjugular intrahepatic portosystemic shunt HE (post-TIPS-HE) can occur as high as 50% of patients with TIPS.
- Post-TIPS-HE can be effectively treated with TIPS reduction or occlusion.

INTRODUCTION

Hepatic encephalopathy (HE) is a devastating neuropsychiatric complication of liver disease that occurs in up to 50% of patients with cirrhosis.[1,2] Alongside ascites, jaundice, and variceal hemorrhage, HE indicates hepatic decompensation and is an independent risk factor for mortality in patients with liver failure.[1,3] HE significantly impairs patient independence and quality of life, even when patients do not have overt symptoms, making it unique when compared with other symptoms of liver failure.[4] The incidence rate of HE is 11.6 per 100 person-years in Medicare enrollees in

[a] Division of Interventional Radiology, Department of Radiology, UCLA Medical Center, David Geffen School of Medicine at UCLA, Los Angeles, CA, USA; [b] Division of Liver and Pancreas Transplant Surgery, Department of Surgery, UCLA Medical Center, David Geffen School of Medicine at UCLA, Los Angeles, CA, USA; [c] Department of Anesthesiology, UCLA Medical Center, David Geffen School of Medicine at UCLA, Los Angeles, CA, USA
* Corresponding author. Ronald Reagan Medical Center at UCLA, David Geffen School of Medicine at UCLA, 757 Westwood Plaza, Suite 2125, Los Angeles, CA 90095-743730
E-mail address: EdwardLee@mednet.ucla.edu

Clin Liver Dis 28 (2024) 317–329
https://doi.org/10.1016/j.cld.2024.01.008
1089-3261/24/© 2024 Elsevier Inc. All rights reserved.
liver.theclinics.com

the United States, and of those, 75,000 to 105,000 patients are hospitalized with HE each year with a 10% to 15% hospital mortality rate.[5–7] This not only provides significant risk for patients with HE who require frequent hospitalization but also incurs a large cost on the US health-care system.[5] Fortunately, new developments in medical management, surgical techniques, and interventional radiology (IR) management have drastically improved outcomes for these patients. In our comprehensive review, we present IR treatment options of 2 notable causes of refractory HE caused by spontaneous portosystemic shunts (SPSS) and transjugular intrahepatic portosystemic shunt (TIPS).

PATHOPHYSIOLOGY OF HEPATIC ENCEPHALOPATHY

Although the exact mechanism of HE is unclear, evidence suggests that it results from impaired metabolism, and excess shunting of ammonia and other gastrointestinal-derived toxins (GITx) through spontaneous or procedurally created portosystemic shunts.[8] Symptoms of HE include impaired memory, cognition, personality, and motor and sensory functions.[3,9] Presentation of HE ranges from mild HE (MHE) to overt HE (OHE) and severity depends on serum levels of ammonia and cerebral edema.[3,10] Although MHE causes few to no recognizable clinical symptoms and requires psychometric testing for detection, OHE presents with observable neurologic and neuropsychiatric symptoms.[11] Both are highly prevalent because 45% of patients with decompensated cirrhosis develop OHE and up to 80% of patients with compensated cirrhosis develop MHE.[1] HE is an independent risk factor for mortality in patients with end-stage liver disease (ESLD), and mortality occurs in up to 15% of in-hospital cases.[3,5,7] A prospective trial demonstrated that, even MHE, which was confirmed on psychometric testing and electroencephalogram, significantly impaired daily functioning when compared with healthy patients.[4]

Cirrhosis, which impairs the metabolism of ammonia, causes most HE cases. However, HE also may occur, by a similar mechanism, secondary to acute liver injuries caused by acute hepatitis and alcohol or drug toxicity.[9,12,13] In acute and chronic liver failure, hepatocytes lose their ability to detoxify portal blood.[1] HE also follows secondary causes, such as infection, dehydration, electrolyte disturbances, or gastrointestinal bleeding, which increase serum ammonia levels.[1,3,14,15] Infection and gastrointestinal bleeding precede approximately 80% of OHE cases.[2] Often, treatment of these precipitating factors will resolve HE. However, many patients with cirrhosis who already have limited liver function will require both acute and maintenance pharmacologic therapy to manage these episodes and prevent recurrence.

Alternatively, the portal venous system can develop collateral vessels that bypass the liver altogether. This occurs via SPSS that bypass the liver and deliver toxic metabolites into systemic circulation, compounding the buildup of ammonia and other GITx already present in liver failure.[11] These shunts (**Table 1**) occur in up to 60% of patients with cirrhosis and commonly arise via connections between the splenic vein and the renal vein (splenorenal shunt), the inferior vena cava (IVC) and the splenic vein (splenocaval shunt), the gastric veins (GV) and left renal vein (gastrorenal shunt), or recanalized paraumbilical veins.[16–18] These shunts can also occur in the absence of liver disease and cause HE.[19] The incidence of HE in patients with SPSS ranges from 48% to 52% in large SPSS (>8 mm) and 34% to 44% in small SPSS (<8 mm).[20] Spontaneous portosystemic shunt-related HE (SPSS-HE) can be treated medically using lactulose and rifaximin. Uniquely, SPSS-HE can also be treated with a minimally invasive procedure such as shunt embolization. This interventional treatment will be discussed later in detail.

Table 1
A summary of spontaneous portosystemic shunts

SPSS	Afferent (Feeding) Vessel	Efferent (Draining) Vessel	Frequency	Note
Splenorenal shunt	Splenic vein branches	Left renal vein	***	Most common cause of SPSS-HE
Spleno-iliac shunts	Splenic vein branches	Iliofemoral vein	**	
Gastro-Azygous shunt (esophageal varices)	GV: Left GV	Azygous and hemiazygous veins	***	Most common cause of esophageal varices
Gastrorenal shunt	GV: Short GV or Posterior GV	Left renal vein	***	Most common cause of gastric variceal bleed
Gastrocaval shunt	GV: Short GV or Posterior GV	IVC	*	Via gastric varices
Left porto-iliac shunts (Paraumbilical vein)	Left portal vein	Iliofemoral veins	***	Common occult cause of HE
Porto-iliac shunts	Main portal vein	Iliofemoral veins	*	—
Meso-renal shunts	SMV or IMV branches	Left renal vein	**	—
Meso-caval shunts	SMV or IMV branches	IVC	*	—

Abbreviations: GV, gastric vein; HE, hepatic encephalopathy; IMV, inferior mesenteric vein; IVC, inferior vena cava; SMV, superior mesenteric vein.
Frequency: ***, very common; **, moderately common; *, least common.

Besides SPSS-HE, iatrogenic portosystemic shunt such as TIPS can cause clinically significant, medically refractory HE. Similar to SPSS, TIPS can bypass as high as 70% to 80% of portal flow, and hence, it increases nonfiltered ammonia and GITx to cause HE. Post-TIPS HE can occur as high as 50% of the patients with TIPS.[21–28] Post-TIPS HE can be treated medically or procedurally. This will be further discussed in the later section.

The definitive treatment of HE from chronic liver failure is liver transplantation.[10] Before the development of model for end-stage liver disease (MELD) based scoring systems, the development of HE alone could qualify patients for liver transplantation.[29,30] Improvements in liver transplantation and candidate selection have drastically improved survival for patients with liver failure.[11,30] Furthermore, although, grade 3 and 4 HE previously resulted in mortality in up to 90% of patients with acute liver failure, liver transplant has drastically improved these outcomes.[9] Liver transplantation has excellent survival and quality of life with 90% and 75% of patients surviving 1 and 5 years, respectively.[9] Unfortunately, due to transplant criteria, social factors, and donor liver availability, many patients are excluded from this life-saving treatment. For those who are waiting for liver transplant or not able to receive a transplant, additional treatment options are necessary to treat refractory HE in patients with chronic ESLDs to improve survival and quality of life. In the next 2 sections, 2 IR procedures for the treatment of HE are discussed in detail.

TREATMENT OF REFRACTORY HE DUE TO SPSS (SPONTANEOUS PORTOSYSTEMIC SHUNT-RELATED HE)
Spontaneous Portosystemic Shunt

Before performing an IR procedure for HE, obtaining cross-sectional imaging with dual or triple phase computed tomography or MRI is critical for successful obliteration of SPSS. The preprocedural imaging can confirm the presence, location, complexity and size of the shunt. Based on the shunt information, a proper size of embolic material can be selected.[31] SPSS occur in several locations and all have some key defining factors (see **Table 1**).[18] For example, gastrorenal shunts occur in approximately 80% to 85% of patients with GV yet are only present in 10% of the total cirrhotic population. Gastrorenal shunts carry a risk for GV bleeding, HE, and less commonly portal vein thrombosis (PVT).[18] Direct splenorenal shunts connect the splenic vein directly to the renal vein and are not associated with gastric varices.[18] These varices are typically only associated with HE and PVT.[18] Other SPSS include those listed in **Table 1**.[18] Although many of these anatomic variants are exceedingly rare, thorough examination of cross-sectional imaging ensures adequate response to and eligibility for IR procedures for HE.[18]

Antegrade Transvenous Obliteration or Retrograde Transvenous Obliteration

For patients who fail medical therapy and are not eligible for transplantation, obliteration of SPSS can reduce systemic ammonia or GITx load.[32] These treatments include transhepatic or transsplenic antegrade transvenous occlusion (eg, antegrade transvenous obliteration [ATO] or transfemoral or transjugular retrograde transvenous obliteration [RTO]) of SPSS.[32,33] Although these interventions were initially created for the management of gastric variceal bleeding, a growing body of evidence supports their use for the management of SPSS-HE, and both procedures can effectively treat acute and chronic episodes of HE.[9,32–37]

In ATO, a direct percutaneous access of portal venous system via transsplenic or transhepatic route is performed. Then, the afferent (feeding) vessels of SPSS at the portal venous system (eg, short GV or superior mesenteric vein branches) are identified and embolized using various embolic and occlusive materials including balloon, coils, plug, glue, gelfoam, and sclerosing agents (**Fig. 1**A). Of note, ATO carries a higher risk for periprocedural bleeding as ATO access requires transhepatic or transsplenic route, which may increase the risk of bleeding, especially for patients who have poor liver synthetic function and coagulopathy.[9] In patients with SPSS-HE with complex systemic shunt and collaterals, RTO may not be technically feasible and ATO may be a preferred method of embolizing SPSS.

RTO can access the efferent (draining) vessels of SPSS at the systemic vein (eg, gastro-renal shunt or spleno-renal shunt) via a femoral or jugular venous route (**Fig. 1**B). This is considered a safer approach because no hepatic or splenic parenchyma and capsule are traversed during the access. Then, RTO retrogradely occludes SPSS, reducing hepatofugal shunt flow, and increasing portal venous flow toward the liver.[38] The RTO can be performed using a balloon with sclerosing agents in a conventional balloon-occluded retrograde transvenous obliteration (BRTO, **Fig. 2**A), coils with gelfoam in coil-assisted retrograde transvenous obliteration (CARTO, **Fig. 2**B) and plugs with gelfoam in plug-assisted retrograde transvenous obliteration (PARTO, **Fig. 2**C). In BRTO, the occlusion balloon is inflated, and sclerosants (ethanolamine oleate or sodium tetradecyl sulfate) are injected distal to the balloon, toward the portal vein.[35] In CARTO and PARTO, a prothrombotic agent, namely gelfoam, rather than sclerosants, is used.[39] With a complete occlusion of SPSS, ATO or RTO can reduce the shunting of ammonia and GITx. It may, however, exacerbate portal hypertension and increase the risk for ascites, variceal hemorrhage, development of new collaterals and PVT.[40–42]

For BRTO, several case reports and case series reported near complete resolution of HE with minimal side effects after BRTO.[34,41,43] A meta-analysis of more than 1000 patients who underwent BRTO before 2012 identified 20 patients who received BRTO for HE or variceal hemorrhage and HE.[44] All 20 of these patients had improvement in HE after treatment.[44] Fukuda and colleagues reported a cohort of 27, all of whom had improvement in HE after 4 months, despite several needing up to 3 treatment sessions.[45] The disadvantages of BRTO is that sclerosants take at least 2 hours (up to 36 hours) to work effectively, and therefore, patients will require an indwelling balloon during treatment for several hours, requiring ICU or high level of care monitoring. It can

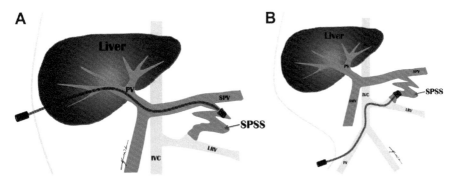

Fig. 1. An illustration comparing the technical approach of ATO to RTO. (*A*) ATO uses a direct percutaneous transhepatic or transsplenic access into the portal venous system. Then, the embolic materials are deployed in the afferent (or feeding) vein of SPSS. (*B*) RTO uses an indirect, systemic (femoral or jugular) venous access into the efferent (or draining) vein of SPSS. Then, the embolic materials are used to occlude the distal end of SPSS.

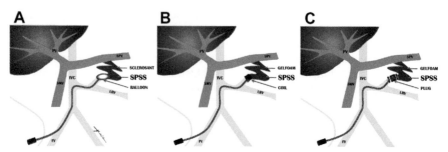

Fig. 2. An illustration of BRTO, CARTO, and PARTO in treating HE. (*A*) BRTO uses a balloon to occlude the efferent (draining) vein of SPSS. Then, a sclerosant is injected retrogradely into the SPSS. (*B*) CARTO and (*C*) PARTO replaces a balloon with embolization coils or vascular plug, respectively, to occlude the SPSS with or without using gelfoam as a thrombogenic agent.

also cause significant discomfort and increasing the risk of treatment failure. Moreover, if the balloon ruptures, the injected sclerosant can rapidly leak and migrate to the pulmonary arteries, leading to respiratory distress and pulmonary embolism.[46] Other reports describe fever, hematuria, pleural effusion, PVT, renal vein thrombosis, pulmonary embolism, ascites, development of new varices, and renal failure in patients who undergo successful BRTO with or without balloon rupture.[40,47]

CARTO and PARTO are modified versions of BRTO that use coils or vascular plugs instead of balloon, and use a gelfoam slurry in place of sclerosants.[33,36,39,48,49] Although these treatments are similar in technique, CARTO and PARTO do not require an indwelling inflated balloon, so these cases are often much shorter and safer. Both treatments are relatively new, and there are several key differences in long-term outcomes. Gwon and colleagues originally reported a retrospective cohort of 7 patients who underwent PARTO for treatment of GV and HE in which HE completely resolved in 7 patients after optimal medical management had previously failed.[36] The same group later reported a multicentered study in which the clinical success rate of treating HE with PARTO was 100% successful in 16 patients.[48] However, the development of collaterals in these patients was first reported by Park and colleagues in which a patient was asymptomatic immediately after PARTO but developed a new or enlarged splenocaval shunt and various collateral shunts 5 months after treatment that led to a recurrence of HE.[49] This case required repeat embolization of these shunts with a combination of plugs, coils, and gelfoam.[49] Kim and colleagues confirmed these findings in an RCT that compared PARTO with BRTO, describing a higher rate of recurrence of GV and recanalization of SPSS in patients who received PARTO.[31]

In 2018, Lee and colleagues examined the use of CARTO as an alternative to BRTO/PARTO in a retrospective review of 43 patients who had a West Haven (WH) score of 2 to 4, and Type C HE who received CARTO (**Fig. 3**).[39] They reported a clinical success rate of 91%.[39] Median WH score improved from 3 to 1, and nearly 70% of patients were completely asymptomatic after treatment.[39] They have noted that few patients without HE improvement after CARTO had incomplete occlusion of the shunt.[39] Consequently, whenever possible, operators should target complete stasis.[39] An extensive collateral vessel network can prevent the use of gelfoam in CARTO. Furthermore, these cases had higher rates of OHE and HE recurrence. Therefore, patients with extensive collateral vessels who do not receive gelfoam during CARTO, should receive close monitoring in the perioperative time period.[39] This study also reported similar rates of ascites, new varices, worsened varices, or bleeding varices after

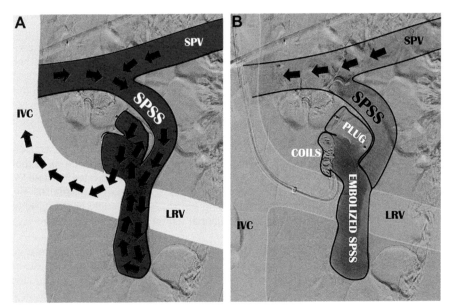

Fig. 3. An illustration and angiographic image of how portal flow changes pre-RTO and post-RTO in treating HE. (*A*) In patients with SPSS-HE, portal venous blood from the splenic vein/portal vein carrying a high concentration of ammonia and other DITx bypasses the liver and shunts into the systemic venous system, such as the left renal vein (*arrows*) via SPSS. (*B*) Once RTO is performed (in this case, both coils and plugs are used), the SPSS is completely obliterated, the portal venous blood is redirected toward the liver, and ammonia or other DITx are no longer shunting into the systemic venous system. These flow dynamic changes improve patients' HE symptoms.

CARTO when compared with previous studies that examined BRTO and PARTO (39.6%).[39] Only 2.3% of patients with these complications required additional intervention through 2 years of follow-up.[39] Lee and colleagues concluded that CARTO is both safe and effective when treating OHE but is limited in cases with extensive collateral vessels that prevent complete occlusion of the shunt.

Interestingly, many of these studies, including those by Laleman and colleagues, and Lee and colleagues, performed receiver-operating characteristic curves and Youden's analysis to examine the impact of MELD scores on survivability after RTO procedures.[39,50] Laleman and colleagues recommended a cutoff of 11, whereas Lee and colleagues recommended that survival is best with a pre-CARTO MELD of less than or equal to 15.[39,50] These scores had similar specificity ($\sim$77%), whereas Lee and colleagues reported a much higher sensitivity of 82.4%, compared with 68.4%.[39,50] Both studies demonstrated that MELD, and, by proxy liver function, should improve after RTO and may even serve as a marker for successful procedural outcome at 1 and 3-month follow-up.[39,50] Inclusion of these criteria in future studies can help to identify which patients will benefit most from RTO.

TREATMENT OF REFRACTORY HE DUE TO TRANSJUGULAR INTRAHEPATIC PORTOSYSTEMIC SHUNT

TIPS is a widely accepted treatment option for complications of portal hypertension including refractory ascites and variceal bleeding.[51–53] However, TIPS is associated with several major clinical complications including new or worsened HE. Post-TIPS HE can be extremely devastating for the patients and their family, and it has a high incidence rate as high as 29% to 50%.[21–28] There are several pre-TIPS risk factors associated with post-TIPS HE including high serum total bilirubin level, age greater than 65 years, and elevated serum creatinine level.[21,26,54,55] Interestingly, well-controlled pre-TIPS HE is not considered a significant risk factor for post-TIPS HE,[56] and this is also described in the American Association for the Study of Liver Diseases updated practice guideline that HE is neither an absolute nor a relative contraindication for TIPS placement.[53]

Of those with post-TIPS HE, the majority (up to 90%) of patients can be medically managed. Unfortunately, 8% to 10% of post-TIPS patients may experience HE refractory to medical treatments such as lactulose or rifaximin, and may require multiple ER visits, hospital admission, ICU admission, and intubations. The post-TIPS HE can considerably affect clinical outcomes including transplant candidacy, and quality of life of these patients and may require additional interventional procedures or liver transplant to cure HE.[21,23,24,57]

IR treatment options for post-TIPS HE include (1) a reduction of TIPS diameter to decrease the shunt blood flow and hence, decrease the bypass rate of ammonia or GIT (**Fig. 4**A), and (2) a complete occlusion of TIPS to entirely remove any shunting of ammonia or GIT through TIPS (**Fig. 4**B). Several different methods of TIPS reduction

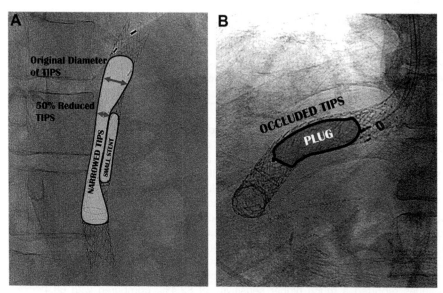

Fig. 4. An illustration and fluoroscopic image of TIPS reduction and TIPS occlusion in the treatment of post-TIPS HE. (*A*) This is an illustration of the parallel stent TIPS reduction technique. In an existing TIPS with a full diameter of 8 or 10 mm causing HE, 2 stents (1 smaller stent and 1 covered stent) are deployed simultaneously in parallel within the existing TIPS stent. This can reduce the TIPS diameter by 40% to 80% and improve patients' HE symptoms. (*B*) If TIPS reduction fails to reverse patients' HE symptoms, TIPS occlusion may be considered. The decision is made in a multidisciplinary meeting. Then, using either a vascular plug or coils, the TIPS is completely occluded. The patients' symptoms may improve after the TIPS is occluded. However, in a small number of cases, TIPS reduction or occlusion may not improve the patient's HE symptoms, and the patient may need a liver transplant to cure.

have been proposed and performed with various clinical success rates of 33% to 100% improvement of post-TIPS HE[21-23,57-62] and complete resolution of HE symptoms in 25% to 80% of patients.[21-24,57,58,60] These clinical improvements after TIPS reduction have been associated with survival rate of 75% in up to 16 months follow-up.[23,24,57,63] As expected, a reversal of TIPS, which was initially performed to treat refractory ascites and variceal bleeding, may cause recurrence of these symptoms as high as 60% and 15%, respectively.[21-24,57,58,60]

Besides treating post-TIPS HE with TIPS reduction or occlusion, some of the recent studies have shown that preventive measures can be implemented before or during TIPS procedures to reduce the post-TIPS HE. In a recent randomized controlled trial, Lv and colleagues demonstrated that embolization of large SPSS during the TIPS procedure in variceal bleeding patients has significantly reduced the risk of overt post-TIPS HE (21.2% vs 48.3%, $P = .043$).[64] In a different recent study, taking 600 mg of rifaximin twice a day before TIPS procedure significantly reduce the rate of post-TIPS HE in alcoholic cirrhosis patients (34% vs 53%, $P = .015$).[65] Although it is a small number of studies, given very limited treatment options are available to treat post-TIPS HE, these preventive methods should be highly considered to reduce post-TIPS HE.

SUMMARY

HE is a serious and potentially fatal complication of liver disease that drastically affects quality of life, mortality, and hospitalization rates. Although medical therapy is highly effective, HE remains a leading cause for hospitalization and morbidity in the United States.[2,5] This results in a significant cost to the US health-care system and accounts for a large percentage of inpatient hospitalizations. Of those, many different etiologies of HE, SPSS-HE, and post-TIPS HE have been effectively treated by interventional radiologists. SPSS-HE can be effectively treated by RTOs (BRTO, CARTO, and PARTO), and post-TIPS HE is routinely treated with TIPS reduction. Both minimally invasive procedures are safe and effective tools for the management of refractory encephalopathy and warrants further investigation.

CONFLICT OF INTEREST

None.

ACKNOWLEDGMENTS

Study concept and design (EWL); acquisition of data (EWL and GPM); analysis and interpretation of data (EWL, JJL, and GPM); drafting of the article (EWL, JJL, and GPM); critical revision of the article for important intellectual content (EWL, JJL, and GPM); statistical analysis (None); obtained funding (None); administrative, technical, or material support and study supervision (EWL).

DISCLOSURE

None.

REFERENCES

1. Frederick RT. Current concepts in the pathophysiology and management of hepatic encephalopathy. Gastroenterol Hepatol 2011;7(4):222–33.
2. Leise MD, Poterucha JJ, Kamath PS, et al. Management of hepatic encephalopathy in the hospital. Mayo Clin Proc 2014;89(2):241–53.

3. Poh Z, Chang P. A current review of the diagnostic and treatment strategies of hepatic encephalopathy. Bangladesh Liver J 2012;2012.

4. Groeneweg M, Quero JC, De Bruijn I, et al. Subclinical hepatic encephalopathy impairs daily functioning. Hepatology 1998;28(1):45–9.

5. Stepanova M, Mishra A, Venkatesan C, et al. In-hospital mortality and economic burden associated with hepatic encephalopathy in the United States from 2005 to 2009. Clin Gastroenterol Hepatol 2012;10(9):1034–41. e1.

6. Tapper EB, Henderson JB, Parikh ND, et al. Incidence of and risk factors for hepatic encephalopathy in a population-based cohort of americans with cirrhosis. Hepatol Commun 2019;3(11):1510–9.

7. Trieu H, Patel A, Wells C, et al. Disparities in mortality and health care utilization for 460,851 hospitalized patients with cirrhosis and hepatic encephalopathy. Dig Dis Sci 2021;66(8):2595–602.

8. McAvoy NC, Hayes PC. Hepatic encephalopathy. Medicine 2007;35(2):108–11.

9. Toris GT, Bikis CN, Tsourouflis GS, et al. Hepatic encephalopathy: an updated approach from pathogenesis to treatment. Med Sci Monit Int Med J Exp Clin Res 2011;17.

10. Vilstrup H, Amodio P, Bajaj J, et al. Hepatic encephalopathy in chronic liver disease: 2014 practice guideline by the American association for the study of liver diseases and the European association for the study of the liver. Hepatology 2014;60.

11. Prakash R, Mullen KD. Mechanisms, diagnosis and management of hepatic encephalopathy. Nat Rev Gastroenterol Hepatol 2010;7(9):515–25.

12. Butterworth RF. Hepatic encephalopathy–a serious complication of alcoholic liver disease. Alcohol Res Health J Natl Inst Alcohol Abus Alcohol 2003;27.

13. Perazzo JC, Tallis S, Delfante A, et al. Hepatic encephalopathy: an approach to its multiple pathophysiological features. World J Hepatol 2012;4.

14. Polson J, Lee WM, American Association for the Study of Liver Disease. AASLD position paper: the management of acute liver failure. Hepatology 2005;41(5): 1179–97.

15. Hassanein TI, Hilsabeck RC, Perry W. Introduction to the hepatic encephalopathy scoring algorithm (HESA). Dig Dis Sci 2008;53(2):529–38.

16. Zardi EM, Uwechie V, Caccavo D, et al. Portosystemic shunts in a large cohort of patients with liver cirrhosis: detection rate and clinical relevance. J Gastroenterol 2009;44(1):76–83.

17. Nardelli S, Riggio O, Turco L, et al. Relevance of spontaneous portosystemic shunts detected with CT in patients with cirrhosis. Radiology 2021;299(1):133–40.

18. Saad WEA. Vascular anatomy and the morphologic and hemodynamic classifications of gastric varices and spontaneous portosystemic shunts relevant to the BRTO procedure. Tech Vasc Intervent Radiol 2013;16(2):60–100.

19. Tanaka H, Saijo Y, Tomonari T, et al. An adult case of congenital extrahepatic portosystemic shunt successfully treated with balloon-occluded retrograde transvenous obliteration. Intern Med 2021;60(12):1839–45.

20. Simon-Talero M, Roccarina D, Martinez J, et al. Association between portosystemic shunts and increased complications and mortality in patients with cirrhosis. Gastroenterology 2018;154(6):1694–1705 e4.

21. Riggio O, Angeloni S, Salvatori FM, et al. Incidence, natural history, and risk factors of hepatic encephalopathy after transjugular intrahepatic portosystemic shunt with polytetrafluoroethylene-covered stent grafts. Am J Gastroenterol 2008;103(11):2738–46.

22. Fanelli F, Salvatori FM, Rabuffi P, et al. Management of refractory hepatic encephalopathy after insertion of TIPS: long-term results of shunt reduction with hourglass-shaped balloon-expandable stent-graft. AJR Am J Roentgenol 2009; 193(6):1696–702.

23. Kochar N, Tripathi D, Ireland H, et al. Transjugular intrahepatic portosystemic stent shunt (TIPSS) modification in the management of post-TIPSS refractory hepatic encephalopathy. Gut 2006;55(11):1617–23.

24. Casadaban LC, Parvinian A, Minocha J, et al. Clearing the confusion over hepatic encephalopathy after tips creation: incidence, prognostic factors, and clinical outcomes. Dig Dis Sci 2015;60(4):1059–66.

25. Nolte W, Wiltfang J, Schindler C, et al. Portosystemic hepatic encephalopathy after transjugular intrahepatic portosystemic shunt in patients with cirrhosis: clinical, laboratory, psychometric, and electroencephalographic investigations. Hepatology 1998;28(5):1215–25.

26. Routhu M, Safka V, Routhu SK, et al. Observational cohort study of hepatic encephalopathy after transjugular intrahepatic portosystemic shunt (TIPS). Ann Hepatol 2017;16(1):140–8.

27. Masson S, Mardini HA, Rose JD, et al. Hepatic encephalopathy after transjugular intrahepatic portosystemic shunt insertion: a decade of experience. QJM 2008; 101(6):493–501.

28. De Keyzer B, Nevens F, Laenen A, et al. Percutaneous shunt reduction for the management of TIPS-induced acute liver decompensation: a follow-up study. Ann Hepatol 2016;15(6):911–7.

29. Kamath PS, Kim WR, Advanced Liver Disease Study Group. The model for end-stage liver disease (MELD). Hepatology 2007;45(3):797–805.

30. Kim WR, Biggins SW, Kremers WK, et al. Hyponatremia and mortality among patients on the liver-transplant waiting list. N Engl J Med 2008;359(10):1018–26.

31. Kim YH, Kim YH, Kim CS, et al. Comparison of balloon-occluded retrograde transvenous obliteration (BRTO) using ethanolamine oleate (EO), BRTO using sodium tetradecyl sulfate (STS) foam and vascular plug-assisted retrograde transvenous obliteration (PARTO). Cardiovasc Intervent Radiol 2016;39.

32. Blei AT, Cordoba J, Practice Parameters Committee of the American College of Gastroenterology. Practice parameters committee of the American college of G. hepatic encephalopathy. Am J Gastroenterol 2001;96.

33. Lee EW, Saab S, Gomes AS, et al. Coil-assisted retrograde transvenous obliteration (CARTO) for the treatment of portal hypertensive variceal bleeding: preliminary results. Clin Transl Gastroenterol 2014;5.

34. Ibukuro K, Sugihara T, Tanaka R, et al. Balloon-occluded retrograde transvenous obliteration (BRTO) for a direct shunt between the inferior mesenteric vein and the inferior vena cava in a patient with hepatic encephalopathy. J Vasc Interv Radiol JVIR 2007;18.

35. Sabri SS, Saad WE. Balloon-occluded retrograde transvenous obliteration (BRTO): technique and intraprocedural imaging. Semin Intervent Radiol 2011;28.

36. Gwon DI, Ko GY, Yoon HK, et al. Gastric varices and hepatic encephalopathy: treatment with vascular plug and gelatin sponge-assisted retrograde transvenous obliteration—a primary report. Radiology 2013;268.

37. Toyonaga A, Oho K. Should B-RTO be the first-line treatment for portosystemic encephalopathy? Intern Med 2001;40.

38. Choi YH, Yoon CJ, Park JH, et al. Balloon-occluded retrograde transvenous obliteration for gastric variceal bleeding: its feasibility compared with transjugular intrahepatic portosystemic shunt. Korean J Radiol 2003;4.

39. Lee EW, Saab S, Kaldas F, et al. Coil-assisted retrograde transvenous obliteration (CARTO): an alternative treatment option for refractory hepatic encephalopathy. Am J Gastroenterol 2018;113.

40. Park JK, Saab S, Kee ST, et al. Balloon-occluded retrograde transvenous obliteration (BRTO) for treatment of gastric varices: review and meta-analysis. Dig Dis Sci 2014;60. https://doi.org/10.1007/s10620-014-3485-8.

41. Baimakhanov Z, Soyama A, Takatsuki M, et al. Effective balloon-occluded retrograde transvenous obliteration of the superior mesenteric vein-inferior vena cava shunt in a patient with hepatic encephalopathy after living donor liver transplantation. Clin J Gastroenterol 2014;7.

42. Saad WE, Sabri SS. Balloon-occluded retrograde transvenous obliteration (BRTO): technical results and outcomes. Semin Intervent Radiol 2011;28.

43. Mukund A, Rajesh S, Arora A, et al. Efficacy of balloon-occluded retrograde transvenous obliteration of large spontaneous lienorenal shunt in patients with severe recurrent hepatic encephalopathy with foam sclerotherapy: initial experience. J Vasc Interv Radiol JVIR 2012;23.

44. Park JK, Saab S, Kee ST, et al. Balloon-occluded retrograde transvenous obliteration (BRTO) for treatment of gastric varices: review and meta-analysis. Dig Dis Sci 2015;60(6):1543–53.

45. Fukuda T, Hirota S, Sugimura K. Long-term results of balloon-occluded retrograde transvenous obliteration for the treatment of gastric varices and hepatic encephalopathy. J Vasc Interv Radiol JVIR 2001;12.

46. Park SJ, Chung JW, Kim H-C, et al. The prevalence, risk factors, and clinical outcome of balloon rupture in balloon-occluded retrograde transvenous obliteration of gastric varices. J Vasc Intervent Radiol 2010;21(4):503–7.

47. Akahoshi T, Hashizume M, Tomikawa M, et al. Long-term results of balloon-occluded retrograde transvenous obliteration for gastric variceal bleeding and risky gastric varices: a 10-year experience. J Gastroenterol Hepatol 2008;23.

48. Gwon DI, Kim YH, Ko G-Y, et al. Vascular plug–assisted retrograde transvenous obliteration for the treatment of gastric varices and hepatic encephalopathy: a prospective multicenter study. J Vasc Intervent Radiol 2015;26(11):1589–95.

49. Park JK, Cho SK, Kee S, Lee EW. Vascular plug-assisted retrograde transvenous obliteration of portosystemic shunts for refractory hepatic encephalopathy: a case report. Case Rep Radiol 2014;2014:391420.

50. Laleman W, Simon-Talero M, Maleux G, et al. Embolization of large spontaneous portosystemic shunts for refractory hepatic encephalopathy: a multicenter survey on safety and efficacy. Hepatology 2013;57.

51. Garcia-Tsao G, Abraldes JG, Berzigotti A, et al. Portal hypertensive bleeding in cirrhosis: risk stratification, diagnosis, and management: 2016 practice guidance by the American Association for the study of liver diseases. Hepatology 2017; 65(1):310–35.

52. Bureau C, Thabut D, Oberti F, et al. Transjugular intrahepatic portosystemic shunts with covered stents increase transplant-free survival of patients with cirrhosis and recurrent ascites. Gastroenterology 2017;152(1):157–63.

53. Boyer TD, Haskal ZJ, American Association for the Study of Liver D. The role of transjugular intrahepatic portosystemic shunt (TIPS) in the management of portal hypertension: update 2009. Hepatology 2010;51(1):306.

54. Suraweera D, Sundaram V, Saab S. Evaluation and management of hepatic encephalopathy: current status and future directions. Gut Liver 2016;10(4):509–19.

55. Guevara M, Baccaro ME, Rios J, et al. Risk factors for hepatic encephalopathy in patients with cirrhosis and refractory ascites: relevance of serum sodium concentration. Liver Int 2010;30(8):1137–42.
56. Saab S, Zhao M, Asokan I, et al. History of hepatic encephalopathy is not a contraindication to transjugular intrahepatic portosystemic shunt placement for refractory ascites. Clin Transl Gastroenterol 2021;12(8):e00378.
57. Maleux G, Verslype C, Heye S, et al. Endovascular shunt reduction in the management of transjugular portosystemic shunt-induced hepatic encephalopathy: preliminary experience with reduction stents and stent-grafts. AJR Am J Roentgenol 2007;188(3):659–64.
58. Cookson DT, Zaman Z, Gordon-Smith J, et al. Management of transjugular intrahepatic portosystemic shunt (TIPS)-associated refractory hepatic encephalopathy by shunt reduction using the parallel technique: outcomes of a retrospective case series. Cardiovasc Intervent Radiol 2011;34(1):92–9.
59. Pereira K, Carrion AF, Salsamendi J, et al. Endovascular management of refractory hepatic encephalopathy complication of transjugular intrahepatic portosystemic shunt (TIPS): comprehensive review and clinical practice algorithm. Cardiovasc Intervent Radiol 2016;39(2):170–82.
60. Monnin-Bares V, Thony F, Sengel C, et al. Stent-graft narrowed with a lasso catheter: an adjustable TIPS reduction technique. J Vasc Intervent Radiol 2010;21(2):275–80.
61. Taylor AG, Kolli KP, Kerlan RK Jr. Techniques for transjugular intrahepatic portosystemic shunt reduction and occlusion. Tech Vasc Intervent Radiol 2016;19(1):74–81.
62. Madoff DC, Wallace MJ, Ahrar K, et al. TIPS-related hepatic encephalopathy: management options with novel endovascular techniques. Radiographics 2004;24(1):21–36, discussion 36-7.
63. Wong RJ, Gish RG, Ahmed A. Hepatic encephalopathy is associated with significantly increased mortality among patients awaiting liver transplantation. Liver Transplant 2014;20(12):1454–61.
64. Lv Y, Chen H, Luo B, et al. Concurrent large spontaneous portosystemic shunt embolization for the prevention of overt hepatic encephalopathy after TIPS: a randomized controlled trial. Hepatology 2022;76(3):676–88.
65. Bureau C, Thabut D, Jezequel C, et al. The use of rifaximin in the prevention of overt hepatic encephalopathy after transjugular intrahepatic portosystemic shunt: a randomized controlled trial. Ann Intern Med 2021;174(5):633–40.

Future Therapies of Hepatic Encephalopathy

Adam P. Buckholz, MD, MS, Robert S. Brown Jr, MD, MPH*

KEYWORDS

- Hepatic encephalopathy • Portal hypertension • Experimental therapeutics
- Disease management

KEY POINTS

- Hepatic Encephalopathy remains a common and highly morbid complication of chronic liver disease.
- There are few current therapies, which are limited especially by patient tolerance and cost.
- As the pathophysiology of encephalopathy becomes better understood, there are multiple promising potential targets for therapeutics.
- This review provides an overview of the emerging therapeutics for hepatic encephalopathy and their relation to pathways of disease.

INTRODUCTION

Hepatic Encephalopathy (HE) is a spectrum of neuropsychiatric disturbances that is a common and highly morbid complication of chronic liver disease. It confers significant reduction in health-related quality of life[1] and is associated with increased mortality overall.[2] In addition, although HE is classically thought to be reversible, emerging evidence suggests that HE has lasting effects on cognition and well-being even after correction of an acute episode.

The classification and varying presentation of HE are beyond the scope of this review; however, it should be noted that HE can arise from various diseases, including acute and chronic liver disease and portosystemic shunting. Likewise, HE can be episodic or persistent and can exist in a spectrum of severities from subtle changes (termed covert encephalopathy) to coma (overt encephalopathy), graded according to the West Haven Criteria.[3] HE is most commonly seen in chronic liver disease, where up to 40% will eventually develop overt disease, and the prevalence of covert HE is greater than 50%.[4] A significant portion of HE is precipitated by an acute destabilizing event, especially in those with cirrhosis; such events include infection, bleeding,

Division of Gastroenterology and Hepatology, New York/Presbyterian-Weill Cornell Medical College, 1305 York Avenue, 4th Floor, New York, NY 10021, USA
* Corresponding author.
E-mail address: Rsb2005@med.cornell.edu

Clin Liver Dis 28 (2024) 331–344
https://doi.org/10.1016/j.cld.2024.02.002
1089-3261/24/© 2024 Elsevier Inc. All rights reserved.
liver.theclinics.com

electrolyte abnormality, constipation, renal failure, sedating medication, or treatment nonadherence.

HE is now thought to have persistent cognitive damage, potentially owing to astrocyte senescence, with research demonstrating that those with HE have worse 1- and 5-year outcomes even after transplant.[5] Early detection and appropriate therapy are therefore crucial, but treatment options remain limited for clinicians. This review briefly discusses the few approved options, before expanding on emerging therapeutics and how they relate to HE pathophysiology.

The pathophysiology of HE is complex and incompletely understood, but the broad overview offered here contextualizes current and proposed therapeutics for HE. Ammonia has long been understood to be a critically important neurotoxic agent in the development of HE.[6] A common inorganic nitrogenous waste, it is produced both by human tissue such as muscle and intestine, and especially, by urease-expressing bacteria in the gut.[7] Reduced hepatic metabolism and shunting owing to portal hypertension lead to drastically increased systemic exposure to ammonia. This ammonia crosses the blood-brain border where it is metabolized by a combination with glutamate-to-glutamine in astrocytes,[8] creating an osmotic gradient with subsequent astrocyte swelling and neuroinflammation.[9] Ammonia and other toxins also potentiate neuroinhibitory cascades and have a direct neurotoxic effect on synaptic transmission.[10,11] In cirrhosis, progressive frailty and reduced muscle mass also deprive patients of an alternative route for ammonia detoxification, and reduced branch chain amino acids in cirrhosis reduce capacity for peripheral glutamine synthesis from ammonia.[12] In addition, systemic inflammation and oxidative stress present in cirrhosis are recognized as significant factors in the pathogenesis of HE. This review focuses on current and emerging treatment options for HE, with a focus on how disease pathophysiology is being addressed by experimental therapeutics (**Fig. 1**).

CURRENT THERAPEUTICS

The nonabsorbable disaccharides lactulose and lactitol have long formed the backbone of HE management.[13] They are metabolized into a short-chain acidic form by gut bacteria and exert their protective effects in multiple ways. First, they increase osmolality of colonic contents, with a laxative effect that decreases colonic transit time and reduces burden of ammonia-genic bacteria. In addition, they reduce the pH of the colonic lumen, promoting conversion of ammonia into the nonabsorbed positively charged ammonium state. The lowering of colonic pH also helps to reduce proliferation of pathogenic bacteria. Usage is most often limited by side effects, including flatulence, abdominal bloating, and diarrhea; nonadherence to lactulose is a key factor in recurrent HE.[14]

The nonabsorbable antibiotic rifaximin inhibits bacterial RNA synthesis[15] and likely has multimodal action in HE improvement. It selectively modulates ammonia production by acting on pathogenic colonic bacteria to reduce efficacy of the RNA polymerase without altering microbiome diversity.[16] It also may help improve gut barrier function, reducing endotoxemia and systemic inflammation.[17] A poorly absorbed antibiotic, it has fewer systemic side effects than other antibiotics that have been previously used in HE, making it a useful agent, especially in recurrent HE.[18] However, its high cost sometimes limits availability.

Finally, standard-of-care management in acute HE entails identifying and correcting underlying exogenous factors, such as infection, bleeding, or electrolyte imbalance. Identifying and correcting such factors may result in up to 90% resolution rate in an

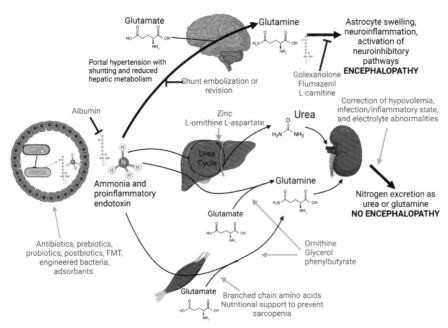

Fig. 1. Nitrogen metabolism in the form of ammonia is a multiorgan process, and increased ammonia exposure in the brain in the setting of cirrhosis and portal hypertension is a major factor in the development of HE. This simplified schematic demonstrates how many experimental therapeutics favor reduced cerebral hyperammonemia and may help treat HE. Created with BioRender.com.

acute episode.[19] Similarly, patients with large portosystemic shunts (either spontaneous[20] or surgical[21]) may benefit from modification, closure, or obliteration.

DISCUSSION ON EMERGING AND EXPERIMENTAL THERAPEUTICS
Albumin

Albumin has established utility in the management of renal insufficiency, overdiuresis, and infection in cirrhosis, all of which can be precipitants of HE. However, because of its known anti-inflammatory properties, as well as studies suggesting that albumin may lower serum ammonia, colloid therapy with albumin has been investigated as a possible treatment or prevention tool in HE. The RELIEF trial demonstrated no improvement in overall outcomes with albumin dialysis, but a trend toward improved HE.[22] When added to lactulose, treatment with albumin improved serum ammonia, inflammatory markers, and proportion of patients with complete HE reversal in a small randomized study by Sharma and colleagues.[23] Although another study by Simón-Talero and colleagues[24] failed to find a clear benefit, a meta-analysis of 12 pooled studies suggested that albumin was associated with decreased risk of HE among those both without prior HE (OR, 0.53; 95% CI, 0.32, 0.86) or prior HE (OR, 0.43; 95% CI, 0.27, 0.68).[25] Finally, a recent randomized double-blind placebo-controlled study of weekly infusions of albumin in outpatients with a history of HE showed reduced cognitive impairment and inflammatory markers with albumin treatment.[26] Despite this, well-controlled studies are lacking at this time, especially to help adjudicate whether the benefit in HE is in fact simply by reversing predisposing factors.

Urea Cycle Modulators

In liver failure and with shunting of portal flow into systemic circulation, the hepatic urea cycle is underused. The urea cycle converts ammonia to urea, primarily in the liver, for excretion in the kidneys, and is the primary source of ammonia disposal in the healthy state.[27] The reduced utilization of the urea cycle owing to hepatic dysfunction and portosystemic shunting results in higher levels of systemic ammonia exposure.

L-ornithine and L-aspartate (LOLA) has been proposed as a method to augment the urea cycle. A mixture of 2 amino acids, LOLA stimulates urea synthesis in periportal hepatocytes and glutamine synthesis in skeletal muscle. A randomized blinded study of 193 patients with acute overt hepatic encephalopathy (OHE) suggested that LOLA reduced recovery time (1.92 vs 2.50 days; $P = .002$) and ammonia levels relative to lactulose and ceftriaxone.[28] In one large Cochrane review and meta-analysis of 36 clinical trials with 2377 participants, LOLA was associated with reduced mortality (RR, 0.42; 95% CI, 0.24, 0.72), but this beneficial effect was not statistically significant when excluding trials with a high risk of bias.[29] This meta-analysis did, however, find that LOLA appeared safe relative to standard-of-care management. The investigators concluded that although it appears LOLA may have a mortality benefit and improve outcomes, higher-quality randomized data are needed before supporting its use, and it remains unavailable in the United States.

Zinc is an important cofactor in the urea cycle, and zinc metabolism impairment and subsequent deficiency are common in cirrhosis.[30] For this reason, and its widespread availability and low expense, supplementation has long been of interest in the management of HE. Unfortunately, small trials, such as a crossover study of 15 participants[31] and a subsequent meta-analysis, have failed to find clear clinical benefit.[32] For this reason, it is not currently considered useful in HE management.

Urinary Ammonia Excretion

The kidneys have net positive ammonia production, with regulation of ammonia excretion a key factor in acid-base homeostasis.[33] In settings of increased acidemia or high ammonia load, healthy kidneys can rapidly upregulate ammonia excretion,[34] and this method of nonurea urinary ammonia excretion takes outsized importance in chronic liver disease. In conditions of hypokalemia and acidosis in chronic liver disease, the kidney also uses glutamine preferentially for potassium recovery in the renal tubules and proton disposal, respectively.[35]

Ornithine phenylacetate is a proposed ammonia scavenger that increases urinary excretion of glutamine in the form of phenylacetylglutamine, preventing it from being used by the kidneys for formation of new ammonia.[36] Although preliminary data suggested that ornithine was effective in lowering serum ammonia,[37] a recent randomized trial failed to demonstrate a statistically significant improvement in time to clinical response, meaning further studies are needed before clinical utilization.[38]

Glycerol phenylbutyrate acts similarly to ornithine phenylacetate, by trapping glutamine for urinary excretion. Already used in genetic urea cycle disorders, it has been shown to reduce serum ammonia levels in small studies.[39] A double-blinded randomized controlled trial of 178 patients with cirrhosis found a reduction in proportion of first-time HE events (21 vs 36%; $P = .02$) and total events (35 vs 57; $P = .04$). As a phase II trial, it was somewhat underpowered but shows promise if studied further.[40]

Antibiotics

Nitazoxanide is an antiprotozoal agent Food and Drug Administration approved for management of diarrheal illnesses. A small head-to-head study comparing twice-daily nitazoxanide with twice-daily rifaximin demonstrated prolonged remission (137 vs 67 days on average; $P<.01$).[41] Despite the promising results, this study conducted in Egypt must be followed by larger controlled studies, with one study currently recruiting (NCT04161053).

Rifaximin soluble solid dispersion (SSD) tablets are a novel preparation to improve delivery and pharmacokinetics of rifaximin therapy. Because of reduced bile acid concentrations in cirrhosis, the largely water-insoluble standard rifaximin formulation may have reduced efficacy compared with a water-soluble formulation (SSD).[42] A recent phase II study of rifaximin SSD in various formulations did not meet its primary endpoint relative to placebo for increased time to hospitalization or all-cause mortality, but in a second trial an immediate release formulation reduced time to OHE recovery.[43] A phase III study is currently planned (NCT05071716).

Microbiome Modulation with 'Biotics (Prebiotics, Probiotics, and Postbiotics)

Endotoxemia and systemic inflammation are integral to development and progression of HE. It is increasingly clear that altered microbiome in those with worsening liver disease contributes to a proinflammatory state.[44] It is widely accepted that the gut microbiome is altered in those with cirrhosis. Subsequent gut translocation potentiates systemic inflammation and is also thought to be a driver of HE development.[45] A lower intestinal pH is unfavorable to the survival of several bacteria known to produce urease, thus increasing ammonia production, including *Klebsiella* and *Proteus*.

Severity of dysbiosis is directly related to severity of liver dysfunction.[46] For this reason, further refinement of microbiome-targeted therapies is a key development opportunity for HE management (**Fig. 2**). Such therapies could target either reduced

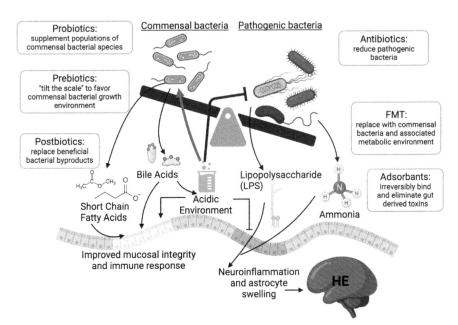

Fig. 2. Progressive dysbiosis and gut membrane dysfunction are now clearly recognized in the pathophysiology of HE. Several experimental therapies in HE address either gut microbial composition or the gut metabolic environment to favor reduced systemic ammonia absorption and gut-induced inflammation. Created with BioRender.com.

inflammation or reduced ammonia load produced by gut bacteria by modulation of relative gut microbial composition. A key study previously demonstrated that reduction of relative *Escherichia coli* and *Staphylococcal* populations in favor of non–urease-producing *Lactobacillus* using probiotics and a prebiotic improved systemic inflammation and covert hepatic encephalopathy (CHE) symptoms.[47]

Prebiotics are nondigestible food products intended to favorably stimulate fermentation and growth of beneficial microorganisms. Lactulose itself is a prebiotic, and its ability to safely modulate ammonia production in the gut has been attractive for HE research. One prebiotic, *Gelsectan*, is derived of mucosal protective agents, such as xyloglucan, with polysaccharides that are thought to promote commensal bacteria and may increase mucosal integrity.[48] It has demonstrated some promise in irritable bowel syndrome, and a clinical trial has been registered to evaluate it in HE (NCT05189834).

Probiotics, which are live micro-organisms that are generally ingested, are a commonly used way to manipulate the microbial composition of the gut. Several strains have been noted in controlled studies to reduce ammonia levels and incidence of overt disease in those with HE. Lactobacillus supplementation, specifically, has been repeatedly demonstrated to be effective at reducing ammonia levels and improving cognitive function, either as an isolated strain or in combination with other bacterial formulations, such as in the *VSL #3*/Visbiome (VSL Pharmaceuticals, Inc/ExeGI Pharma). In one unblinded randomized study, use of VSL #3 reduced the incidence of overt HE episodes in those with cirrhosis.[49] Similar results have been found in other studies and using different strains.

Research thus far has been relatively limited, and a legal dispute between the developer of VSL #3 and the subsequent ownership over a unilateral change in strain composition speaks to the somewhat ephemeral and variable nature of the various brands and strains. A Cochrane review published in 2017 asserted that although probiotics (either in combination with or instead of lactulose) may improve recovery and prevent disease progression, there is no clear impact on mortality.[50] In addition, extant research in this field was thought to be possibly affected by bias and random error. Another limitation to the current use of probiotics is that the exact target population is unclear. In one small study, VSL #3 was found to have more profound protective inflammatory changes in patients with alcohol or metabolic liver disease than in those with cirrhosis owing to hepatitis C.[51] There also may be resistance to long-term colonization and durable uptake of strains not already adapted to the gut environment, limiting use.[52]

One additional limitation of probiotic therapy is that it does not change the host environment (metabolites, gut milieu) that perpetuates dysbiosis in those with cirrhosis. For example, bile acids are an important modulator of the gut microbiome and have decreased concentration in those with advanced liver disease.[53] Potentially by influencing primary and secondary bile acid concentration in the gut, indirect influence on microbial populations could lead to reduced inflammatory markers and improved outcomes in HE.[54]

Other such microbial derived metabolites, often called "*postbiotics*," may eventually have clinical utility either independent of or in combination with classical HE treatment options. These include tryptophan derivatives, short-chain fatty acids, and choline compounds.[55]

Microbial-based therapy not only is confined to the hindgut but also as periodontal treatment has been demonstrated to reduce salivary dysbiosis and improve cognition in those with HE by decreasing endotoxemia and salivary inflammation.[56]

One future avenue for probiotic therapy in HE is the use of *engineered bacteria*, potentially to consume a toxic metabolite, such as ammonia, converting it to a nontoxic byproduct, such as L-arginine.[57] However, the first in-human randomized trial failed to show effective lowering of serum ammonia, making any clinical application some distance away.[58]

Stool-derived Therapies

Fecal microbiota transplantation (FMT) has been demonstrated to improve outcomes in other conditions of significant gut dysbiosis, such as recurrent *Clostridium difficile* infection.[7] FMT involves the transfer of a complete community of gut microorganisms from a donor, with significantly increased diversity over the limited number of strains in a probiotic. This potentially leads to a more comprehensive restoration of gut microbial balance. They also incorporate enzymes and metabolites from the donor stool, above and beyond the transplanted organisms, which may also affect the urea/ammonia cycle. In a seminal study of those with recurrent HE, FMT using a donor specifically selected for high levels of short-chain fatty acid–producing bacteria, such as *Lachnospiraceae*, resulted in improved cognition and reduced hospitalization at 30 days.[59] Interestingly, follow-up in the same group of patients suggested that the population of *Lachnospiraceae* returned to pre-FMT levels, but cognition remained better in the FMT group, and HE hospitalizations remained lower.[60] One limitation to FMT therapy at this juncture is that donor stool characteristics have been shown to influence outcomes, making standardization difficult.[61] Future research will need to better elucidate the appropriate donor profile, as well as the recipients most likely to benefit. An FMT study by Bloom and colleagues[62] in HE demonstrated that the relative concentration of short-chain fatty acid–producing bacteria in donor stool influenced recipient outcome. Finally, the promise of FMT must be balanced with the understood risk of inducing an infection, potentially with a drug-resistant organism, in patients with known immune dysfunction.[63]

This risk of infection and the variability of donor profiles may limit broad uptake of FMT in clinical practice. One ongoing clinical trial (NCT04899115) is evaluating the use of *VE303*, a group of 5 strains of commensal, nonpathogenic *Clostridia* species. These strains are derived from donor stool and manufactured from clonal cell banks to increase standardization and reduce risk of resistant strain infection.[64] A phase II study in VE303 recently demonstrated efficacy in prevention of recurrent *C difficile*.[65]

Similarly, *RBX7455* is a standardized donor-derived live therapeutic bacterial product that has been lyophilized ("freeze-dried") after being obtained in large aliquots from a single donor and tested for viable bacterial content. It has the added benefit of room temperature stability for storage and being available in a pH-resistant capsule. Early studies have been promising in *C difficile* infection,[66] with an early-stage trial enrolling for HE (NCT04155099).

Gut Adsorbents

AST-120 and *Yaq-001* are synthetic carbon-based ingestible microspheres that have been developed to adsorb gut toxins, such as ammonia, and, because they are not absorbed systemically, reduce systemic ammonia levels and inflammation. Although promising data were found in rat models,[67] the largest randomized study of AST-120 found no clinical benefit.[68] A clinical trial of Yaq-001 was terminated because of COVID-19,[69] suggesting it will be some time before this potential therapeutic is ready for routine use in HE.

Neurotransmitter Modulation

The influx of toxins, especially ammonia, through the blood-brain barrier leads to increased neuroinflammation mediated by reactive oxidative species, a critical step in the development of HE. For this reason, modulation at the level of the brain is an attractive target for treatment. Neuroinflammation leads to neurosteroid-induced potentiation of the GABA-A system, which is neuroinhibitory and has negative effects on memory, cognition, vigilance, and sleep.[70] A recently developed GABA-A receptor antagonist, golexanolone (GR3027), is under investigation for possible cognitive benefits in HE. In a small, randomized trial of 45 patients with cirrhosis, golexanolone improved vigilance and some cognitive markers, although further studies will be needed to evaluate its possible use to improve outcomes.[71]

L-carnitine crosses the blood-brain barrier, where it facilitates mitochondrial uptake of acetyl Co-A and stimulates phospholipid synthesis while serving as substrate for cerebral energy production.[72] It also has been postulated to be protective against neuroinflammation by reducing free radical production.[73] In a small randomized double-blinded placebo-controlled trial, L-carnitine supplementation improved quality of life and reduced serum ammonia concentration.[74] Unfortunately, a subsequent Cochrane systematic review found that all 5 trials with 398 patients evaluating L-carnitine use were conducted by the same research group with high potential for bias, with no clear clinical benefit.[75] No clinical trials appear to be currently recruiting.

Flumazenil is a synthetic benzodiazepine antagonist hypothesized to have utility in HE through its modulation of inhibitory GABA-A complex receptors, given the posited increased GABAnergic "tone" in those with HE as a result of ammonia and manganese upregulation.[76] In a randomized, double-blinded placebo-controlled trial of flumazenil versus placebo in patients hospitalized with severe HE, flumazenil improved neurologic score in more patients (14.7% vs 3.8%; $P<.01$).[77] A follow-up meta-analysis, however, found that most of the 14 studies evaluated had significant risk of bias but overall suggested a possible short-term benefit for flumazenil in severe HE without a mortality benefit.[78] Its short-half life and need for intravenous administration limit it to use only in hospitalized patients.

Skeletal Muscle Metabolism

Muscle is an important alternate source of ammonia metabolism, especially in the presence of hepatic dysfunction. In portal hypertension, muscular glutamine synthetase conversion of glutamate and ammonia into glutamine helps compensates for reduced hepatic metabolism.

Branched chain amino acids (BCAAs), typically derived from dietary protein, are important metabolic precursors of glutamate, which as above is crucial for subsequent ammonia metabolism.[79] Transamination in the liver of BCAAs results in glutamate, but a combination of portal hypertension and malnutrition results in relative depletion.[80] Reduced relative BCAA concentration (compared with aromatic amino acids) is also thought to negatively affect neurotransmission in the brain. Accordingly, supplementation with either oral[81] or intravenous[82] BCAAs may be beneficial in HE, especially in those with sarcopenia or nutrition deficiency. Across 16 clinical trials, a Cochrane systematic review and meta-analysis concluded that insufficient evidence was present for mortality benefit, but an overall beneficial effect on HE (RR, 0.76; 95% CI, 0.63–0.92) when combining oral and parenteral studies.[83] Unfortunately, they have not been extensively studied in comparison, or as an adjunct therapy, with standard of care in controlled settings. Several early-phase studies are currently evaluating BCAAs in acute-on-chronic liver failure with HE (eg, NCT05700695), but a published abstract suggested mixed results with early but not sustained improvement.[84] The amino acid mixture AXA1655, a combination of BCAAs and LOLA, was studied, demonstrating increased relative BCAA concentration and reduced ammonia in a small trial (n = 40)[85]; however, a follow-up phase II clinical trial was recently terminated by the sponsoring company (NCT04816916). An additional ongoing study (NCT04096014) is evaluating the use of timed protein supplementation with Ensure in the evenings and in the mornings and its effect on muscle mass and HE.

SUMMARY

As the pathophysiology, predisposing factors, and various clinical presentations of HE become better understood, the need for better and more precise therapeutic options grows. As previously posited,[86] an ideal treatment regimen would take into account individual patient characteristics and directly address the multifactorial nature of HE. In general, the current armamentarium of lactulose and rifaximin addresses only a limited scope of the problem, is not uniformly effective, and may not be right for every situation especially when considering toxicity and cost. Given the vast array of potential alternatives that have been tested or are being studied, the future of HE management is potentially bright. It is critically important that well-controlled prospective studies be funded in these areas in order to improve outcomes, while considering additional factors, such as muscle, renal, and neurologic drivers of disease.

CLINICS CARE POINTS

- Lactulose and rifaximin remain the backbone of HE therapy but emerging therapeutics may help close the care gaps that remain.
- In particular, microbiota derived therapies including FMT have shown promise but still require standardization and have limitations including risk of accidental infection.
- While urea cycle modulators such as Zinc and L-ornithine and L-aspartate are fairly low risk, they have repeatedly failed to demonstrate significant advances over current standard therapies, limiting their usefullness.

DISCLOSURE

The authors have nothing to disclose.

REFERENCES

1. Montagnese S, Bajaj JS. Impact of hepatic encephalopathy in cirrhosis on quality-of-life issues. Drugs 2019;79(Suppl 1):11.
2. Bohra A, Worland T, Hui S, et al. Prognostic significance of hepatic encephalopathy in patients with cirrhosis treated with current standards of care. World J Gastroenterol 2020;26(18):2221–31.
3. Weissenborn K. Hepatic encephalopathy: definition, clinical grading and diagnostic principles. Drugs 2019;79(1):5–9.
4. Das A, Dhiman RK, Saraswat VA, et al. Prevalence and natural history of subclinical hepatic encephalopathy in cirrhosis. J Gastroenterol Hepatol 2001;16(5): 531–5.
5. Wong RJ, Aguilar M, Gish RG, et al. The impact of pretransplant hepatic encephalopathy on survival following liver transplantation. Liver Transpl 2015;21(7): 873–80.
6. Shawcross DL, Olde Damink SWM, Butterworth RF, et al. Ammonia and hepatic encephalopathy: the more things change, the more they remain the same. Metab Brain Dis 2005;20(3):169–79.

7. Butterworth RF, Giguère JF, Michaud J, et al. Ammonia: key factor in the pathogenesis of hepatic encephalopathy. Neurochem Pathol 1987;6(1–2):1–12.

8. Norenberg MD. Astroglial dysfunction in hepatic encephalopathy. Metab Brain Dis 1998;13(4):319–35.

9. Jayakumar AR, Rao KVR, Schousboe A, et al. Glutamine-induced free radical production in cultured astrocytes. Glia 2004;46(3):296–301.

10. Felipo V, Butterworth RF. Neurobiology of ammonia. Prog Neurobiol 2002;67(4): 259–79.

11. Szerb JC, Butterworth RF. Effect of ammonium ions on synaptic transmission in the mammalian central nervous system. Prog Neurobiol 1992;39(2):135–53.

12. Lattanzi B, D'Ambrosio D, Merli M. Hepatic encephalopathy and sarcopenia: two faces of the same metabolic alteration. J Clin Exp Hepatol 2019;9(1):125–30.

13. Bircher J, Müller J, Guggenheim P, et al. Treatment of chronic portal-systemic encephalopathy with lactulose. Lancet 1966;1(7443):890–2.

14. Chow KW, Ibrahim BM, Yum JJ, et al. Barriers to lactulose adherence in patients with cirrhosis and hepatic encephalopathy. Dig Dis Sci 2023;68(6). https://doi. org/10.1007/S10620-023-07935-Z.

15. Gerard L, Garey KW, DuPont HL. Rifaximin: a nonabsorbable rifamycin antibiotic for use in nonsystemic gastrointestinal infections. Expert Rev Anti Infect Ther 2014;3(2):201–11.

16. Yu X, Jin Y, Zhou W, et al. Rifaximin modulates the gut microbiota to prevent hepatic encephalopathy in liver cirrhosis without impacting the resistome. Front Cell Infect Microbiol 2022;11:1427.

17. Patel VC, Lee S, McPhail MJW, et al. Rifaximin-α reduces gut-derived inflammation and mucin degradation in cirrhosis and encephalopathy: RIFSYS randomised controlled trial. J Hepatol 2022;76(2):332–42.

18. Eltawil KM, Laryea M, Peltekian K, et al. Rifaximin vs conventional oral therapy for hepatic encephalopathy: a meta-analysis. World J Gastroenterol : WJG 2012; 18(8):767.

19. Strauss E, Tramote R, Silva EPS, et al. Double-blind randomized clinical trial comparing neomycin and placebo in the treatment of exogenous hepatic encephalopathy. Hepato-Gastroenterology 1992;39(6):542–5. https://europepmc. org/article/med/1483668.

20. Laleman W, Simon-Talero M, Maleux G, et al. Embolization of large spontaneous portosystemic shunts for refractory hepatic encephalopathy: a multicenter survey on safety and efficacy. Hepatology 2013;57(6):2448–57.

21. Kochar N, Tripathi D, Ireland H, et al. Transjugular intrahepatic portosystemic stent shunt (TIPSS) modification in the management of post-TIPSS refractory hepatic encephalopathy. Gut 2006;55(11):1617.

22. Bañares R, Nevens F, Larsen FS, et al. Extracorporeal albumin dialysis with the molecular adsorbent recirculating system in acute-on-chronic liver failure: the RELIEF trial. Hepatology 2013;57(3):1153–62.

23. Sharma BC, Singh J, Srivastava S, et al. Randomized controlled trial comparing lactulose plus albumin versus lactulose alone for treatment of hepatic encephalopathy. J Gastroenterol Hepatol 2017;32(6):1234–9.

24. Simón-Talero M, García-Martínez R, Torrens M, et al. Effects of intravenous albumin in patients with cirrhosis and episodic hepatic encephalopathy: a randomized double-blind study. J Hepatol 2013;59(6):1184–92.

25. Teh KB, Loo JH, Tam YC, et al. Efficacy and safety of albumin infusion for overt hepatic encephalopathy: a systematic review and meta-analysis. Dig Liver Dis 2021;53(7):817–23.

26. Fagan A, Gavis EA, Gallagher ML, et al. A double-blind randomized placebo-controlled trial of albumin in outpatients with hepatic encephalopathy: HEAL study. J Hepatol 2023;78(2):312–21.
27. Adeva MM, Souto G, Blanco N, et al. Ammonium metabolism in humans. Metabolism 2012;61(11):1495–511.
28. Sidhu SS, Sharma BC, Goyal O, et al. L-ornithine L-aspartate in bouts of overt hepatic encephalopathy. Hepatology 2018;67(2):700–10.
29. Goh ET, Stokes CS, Sidhu SS, et al. L-ornithine L-aspartate for prevention and treatment of hepatic encephalopathy in people with cirrhosis. Cochrane Database Syst Rev 2018;2018(5):CD012410.
30. Himoto T, Masaki T. Associations between zinc deficiency and metabolic abnormalities in patients with chronic liver disease. Nutrients 2018;10(1). https://doi.org/10.3390/NU10010088.
31. Riggio O, Ariosto F, Merli M, et al. Short-term oral zinc supplementation does not improve chronic hepatic encephalopathy. Results of a double-blind crossover trial. Dig Dis Sci 1991;36(9):1204–8.
32. Shen YC, Chang YH, Fang CJ, et al. Zinc supplementation in patients with cirrhosis and hepatic encephalopathy: a systematic review and meta-analysis. Nutr J 2019;18(1). https://doi.org/10.1186/S12937-019-0461-3.
33. Weiner ID, Verlander JW. Renal ammonia metabolism and transport. Compr Physiol 2013;3(1):201.
34. Dejong CHC, Deutz NEP, Soeters PB. Renal ammonia and glutamine metabolism during liver insufficiency-induced hyperammonemia in the rat. J Clin Invest 1993;92(6):2834–40.
35. Gabuzda GJ, Hall PW. Relation of potassium depletion to renal ammonium metabolism and hepatic coma. Medicine 1966;45(6):481–90.
36. Ventura-Cots M, Arranz JA, Simón-Talero M, et al. Safety of ornithine phenylacetate in cirrhotic decompensated patients: an open-label, dose-escalating, single-cohort study. J Clin Gastroenterol 2013;47(10):881–7.
37. Ventura-Cots M, Concepción M, Arranz JA, et al. Impact of ornithine phenylacetate (OCR-002) in lowering plasma ammonia after upper gastrointestinal bleeding in cirrhotic patients. Therap Adv Gastroenterol 2016;9(6):823–35.
38. Rahimi RS, Safadi R, Thabut D, et al. Efficacy and safety of ornithine phenylacetate for treating overt hepatic encephalopathy in a randomized trial. Clin Gastroenterol Hepatol 2021;19(12):2626–35.e7.
39. Kortbeek S, Gilkes C, Khan A, et al. Secondary ammonia scavenge with glycerol phenylbutyrate improves hyperammonemia following portosystemic shunting. JPGN Rep 2022;3(3):e210.
40. Rockey DC, Vierling JM, Mantry P, et al. Randomized, double-blind, controlled study of glycerol phenylbutyrate in hepatic encephalopathy. Hepatology 2014;59(3):1073–83.
41. Glal KAM, Abd-Elsalam SM, Mostafa TM. Nitazoxanide versus rifaximin in preventing the recurrence of hepatic encephalopathy: a randomized double-blind controlled trial. J Hepatobiliary Pancreat Sci 2021;28(10):812–24.
42. Darkoh C, Lichtenberger LM, Ajami N, et al. Bile acids improve the antimicrobial effect of rifaximin. Antimicrob Agents Chemother 2010;54(9):3618–24.
43. Bajaj JS, Hassanein TI, Pyrsopoulos NT, et al. Dosing of rifaximin soluble solid dispersion tablets in adults with cirrhosis: 2 randomized, placebo-controlled trials. Clin Gastroenterol Hepatol 2022;21(3):723–31.e9.
44. Qin N, Yang F, Li A, et al. Alterations of the human gut microbiome in liver cirrhosis. Nature 2014;513(7516):59–64.

45. Fukui H. Role of gut dysbiosis in liver diseases: what have we learned so far? Diseases 2019;7(4):58.
46. Wang J, Wang Y, Zhang X, et al. Gut microbial dysbiosis is associated with altered hepatic functions and serum metabolites in chronic hepatitis B patients. Front Microbiol 2017;8(NOV):2222.
47. Liu Q, Duan ZP, Ha DK, et al. Synbiotic modulation of gut flora: effect on minimal hepatic encephalopathy in patients with cirrhosis. Hepatology 2004;39(5): 1441–9.
48. Trifan A, Burta O, Tiuca N, et al. Efficacy and safety of Gelsectan for diarrhoea-predominant irritable bowel syndrome: a randomised, crossover clinical trial. United European Gastroenterol J 2019;7(8):1093.
49. Lunia MK, Sharma BC, Sharma P, et al. Probiotics prevent hepatic encephalopathy in patients with cirrhosis: a randomized controlled trial. Clin Gastroenterol Hepatol 2014;12(6). https://doi.org/10.1016/J.CGH.2013.11.006.
50. Dalal R, Mcgee RG, Riordan SM, et al. Probiotics for people with hepatic encephalopathy. Cochrane Database Syst Rev 2017;2017(2). https://doi.org/10.1002/14651858.CD008716.PUB3.
51. Loguercio C, Federico A, Tuccillo C, et al. Beneficial effects of a probiotic VSL#3 on parameters of liver dysfunction in chronic liver diseases. J Clin Gastroenterol 2005;39(6):540–3.
52. Fehervari Z. Mechanisms of colonization resistance. Nature Research 2021;. https://www.nature.com/articles/d42859-019-00018-y. [Accessed 8 June 2023].
53. Kakiyama G, Pandak WM, Gillevet PM, et al. Modulation of the fecal bile acid profile by gut microbiota in cirrhosis. J Hepatol 2013;58(5):949.
54. Schwabl P, Hambruch E, Seeland BA, et al. The FXR agonist PX20606 ameliorates portal hypertension by targeting vascular remodelling and sinusoidal dysfunction. J Hepatol 2017;66(4):724–33.
55. Bajaj JS, Ng SC, Schnabl B. Promises of microbiome-based therapies. J Hepatol 2022;76(6):1379.
56. Bajaj JS, Matin P, White MB, et al. Periodontal therapy favorably modulates the oral-gut-hepatic axis in cirrhosis. Am J Physiol Gastrointest Liver Physiol 2018; 315(5):G824–37.
57. Kurtz CB, Millet YA, Puurunen MK, et al. An engineered E. coli Nissle improves hyperammonemia and survival in mice and shows dose-dependent exposure in healthy humans. Sci Transl Med 2019;11(475). https://doi.org/10.1126/SCITRANSLMED.AAU7975.
58. Safety, tolerability and pharmacodynamics of SYNB1020 - study results - ClinicalTrials.gov. https://clinicaltrials.gov/ct2/show/results/NCT03447730?term=SYNB1020&rank=2. [Accessed 3 June 2023].
59. Bajaj JS, Kassam Z, Fagan A, et al. Fecal microbiota transplant from a rational stool donor improves hepatic encephalopathy: a randomized clinical trial. Hepatology 2017;66(6):1727.
60. Bajaj JS, Fagan A, Gavis EA, et al. Long-term outcomes after fecal microbiota transplant in cirrhosis. Gastroenterology 2019;156(6):1921.
61. Moayyedi P, Surette MG, Kim PT, et al. Fecal microbiota transplantation induces remission in patients with active ulcerative colitis in a randomized controlled trial. Gastroenterology 2015;149(1):102–9.e6.
62. Bloom PP, Donlan J, Torres Soto M, et al. Fecal microbiota transplant improves cognition in hepatic encephalopathy and its effect varies by donor and recipient. Hepatol Commun 2022;6(8):2079.

63. DeFilipp Z, Bloom PP, Torres Soto M, et al. Drug-resistant E. coli bacteremia transmitted by fecal microbiota transplant. N Engl J Med 2019;381(21):2043–50.

64. Dsouza M, Menon R, Crossette E, et al. Colonization of the live biotherapeutic product VE303 and modulation of the microbiota and metabolites in healthy volunteers. Cell Host Microbe 2022;30(4):583–98.e8.

65. Louie T, Golan Y, Khanna S, et al. VE303, a defined bacterial consortium, for prevention of recurrent clostridioides difficile infection: a randomized clinical trial. JAMA 2023;329(16):1356–66.

66. Khanna S, Pardi DS, Jones C, et al. RBX7455, a non-frozen, orally administered investigational live biotherapeutic, is safe, effective, and shifts patients' microbiomes in a phase 1 study for recurrent clostridioides difficile infections. Clin Infect Dis 2021;73(7):e1613–20.

67. Bosoi CR, Parent-Robitaille C, Anderson K, et al. AST-120 (spherical carbon adsorbent) lowers ammonia levels and attenuates brain edema in bile duct–ligated rats. Hepatology 2011;53(6):1995–2002.

68. Bajaj JS, Sheikh MY, Chojkier M, et al. 190 AST-120 (spherical carbon adsorbent) in covert hepatic encephalopathy: results of the astute trial. J Hepatol 2013; 58:S84.

69. Safety and tolerability of yaq-001 in patients with cirrhosis - full text view - ClinicalTrials.gov. https://clinicaltrials.gov/ct2/show/NCT03202498. [Accessed 11 June 2023].

70. Agusti A, Llansola M, Hernández-Rabaza V, et al. Modulation of GABAA receptors by neurosteroids. A new concept to improve cognitive and motor alterations in hepatic encephalopathy. J Steroid Biochem Mol Biol 2016;160:88–93.

71. Montagnese S, Lauridsen M, Vilstrup H, et al. A pilot study of golexanolone, a new GABA-A receptor-modulating steroid antagonist, in patients with covert hepatic encephalopathy. J Hepatol 2021;75(1):98–107.

72. Malaguarnera M. Acetyl-L-carnitine in hepatic encephalopathy. Metab Brain Dis 2013;28(2):193–9.

73. Rose C, Felipo V. Limited capacity for ammonia removal by brain in chronic liver failure: potential role of nitric oxide. Metab Brain Dis 2005;20(4):275–83.

74. Malaguarnera M, Bella R, Vacante M, et al. Acetyl-L-carnitine reduces depression and improves quality of life in patients with minimal hepatic encephalopathy. Scand J Gastroenterol 2011;46(6):750–9.

75. Martí-Carvajal AJ, Gluud C, Arevalo-Rodriguez I, et al. Acetyl-L-carnitine for patients with hepatic encephalopathy. Cochrane Database Syst Rev 2019;2019(1). https://doi.org/10.1002/14651858.CD011451.PUB2.

76. Ahboucha S, Butterworth RF. The neurosteroid system: implication in the pathophysiology of hepatic encephalopathy. Neurochem Int 2008;52(4–5):575–87.

77. Barbaro G, Di Lorenzo G, Soldini M, et al. Flumazenil for hepatic encephalopathy grade III and IVa in patients with cirrhosis: an Italian multicenter double-blind, placebo-controlled, cross-over study. Hepatology 1998;28(2):374–8.

78. Goh ET, Andersen ML, Morgan MY, et al. Flumazenil versus placebo or no intervention for people with cirrhosis and hepatic encephalopathy. Cochrane Database Syst Rev 2017;2017(7). https://doi.org/10.1002/14651858.CD002798.PUB3.

79. Kawaguchi T, Izumi N, Charlton MR, et al. Branched-chain amino acids as pharmacological nutrients in chronic liver disease. Hepatology 2011;54(3):1063–70.

80. Yamato M, Muto Y, Yoshida T, et al. Clearance rate of plasma branched-chain amino acids correlates significantly with blood ammonia level in patients with liver cirrhosis. Int Hepatol Commun 1995;3(2):91–6.

81. Marchesini G, Dioguardi FS, Bianchi GP, et al. Long-term oral branched-chain amino acid treatment in chronic hepatic encephalopathy. A randomized double-blind casein-controlled trial. The Italian Multicenter Study Group. J Hepatol 1990;11(1):92–101.
82. Naylor CD, O'Rourke K, Detsky AS, et al. Parenteral nutrition with branched-chain amino acids in hepatic encephalopathy. A meta-analysis. Gastroenterology 1989; 97(4):1033–42.
83. Gluud LL, Dam G, Les I, et al. Branched-chain amino acids for people with hepatic encephalopathy. Cochrane Database Syst Rev 2017;5(5). https://doi.org/10.1002/14651858.CD001939.PUB4.
84. Mehtani R, Premkumar M, Garg S, et al. Intravenous branched chain amino acid infusion is associated with early but ill-sustained recovery of overt hepatic encephalopathy in acute-on-chronic liver failure: a pilot protocol. J Clin Exp Hepatol 2022;12:S30.
85. Chakravarthy MV, Neutel J, Confer S, et al. Safety, tolerability, and physiological effects of AXA1665, a novel composition of amino acids, in subjects with Child-Pugh A and B cirrhosis. Clin Transl Gastroenterol 2020;11(8):e00222.
86. Tapper EB, Jiang ZG, Patwardhan VR. Refining the ammonia hypothesis: a physiology-driven approach to the treatment of hepatic encephalopathy. Mayo Clin Proc 2015;90(5):646–58.

Preventing Readmissions for Hepatic Encephalopathy

Salima S. Makhani, MD, MSc[a], Susan Lee, PharmD, MBA[b],
David Bernstein, MD[c],*

KEYWORDS

- Encephalopathy • Cirrhosis • Readmission • Prevention • Rifaximin

KEY POINTS

- Targeted interventons can prevent readmission for hepatic encephalopathy
- Discharge planning prioritizing medication acquisition, follow-up appointments and disease state education can prevent hospital readmission
- Developing a functional patient centered care including specific aspects of post-discharge care can significantly decrease hospital readmission for hepatic encephalopathy

INTRODUCTION

Hepatic encephalopathy is a strong predictor of hospital readmissions in patients with advanced liver disease. Hepatic encephalopathy is a reversible and potentially preventable complication of portal hypertension which can manifest with a wide variety of neuropsychiatric symptoms ranging from mild abnormalities in cognition, memory, and judgment to severe disorientation, coma, and death. The specific mechanism leading to hepatic encephalopathy remains unknown but is associated with elevated serum ammonia levels in a subset of patients. The diagnosis of hepatic encephalopathy is based on the combination of clinical assessments, neuropsychological, and laboratory testing accompanied by the excluding of other causes of altered mental status. The treatment of hepatic encephalopathy consists of initiating therapies to reduce the accumulation of toxins in the blood, following an appropriate diet and, in severe cases, the need for liver transplantation. The overall care centers on the prevention of precipitating factors through a multidisciplinary approach in tandem with the patient and their support system. Given the strong correlation of hepatic encephalopathy and hospital readmissions, targeted interventions to improve management of hepatic encephalopathy from the inpatient to

[a] Zucker School of Medicine at Hofstra/Northwell, 300 Community Drive, Manhasset, NY 11030, USA; [b] Northwell Health Office of Access Strategy, 330 South Service Road, Melville, NY 11747, USA; [c] NYU Grossman School of Medicine, 240 East 38th Street, 23rd Floor, New York, NY 10016, USA
* Corresponding author.
E-mail address: david.bernstein@nyulangone.org

Clin Liver Dis 28 (2024) 345–358
https://doi.org/10.1016/j.cld.2024.01.001
1089-3261/24/© 2024 Elsevier Inc. All rights reserved.

outpatient setting may have the greatest impact on preventing recurrence and readmissions.

IMPACT OF RECURRENT HEPATIC ENCEPHALOPATHY ON THE QUALITY OF LIFE

Recurrent episodes of hepatic encephalopathy in patients are associated with persistent cognitive impairment and reduced quality of life.[1] The recurrent nature can exacerbate the progressive deterioration in cognitive and motor function, leading to the risk of complications, such as falls, infection, malnutrition, and also may impair driving ability.[2] In one study, patients with preoperative, recurrent hepatic encephalopathy experienced persistent cognitive impairment in the form of visuospatial relationships, language, and long-term memory 18-month after liver transplantation.[3]

The cognitive decline in memory, judgment, and comprehension creates challenges for the patient to attend to their activities of daily life. The unpredictability and complexity of this disease makes it difficult for patients' support systems to acknowledge the deterioration of the patient's health, ultimately leading to hospital readmissions in the setting of inadequate education and awareness of monitoring symptoms appropriate in the outpatient setting. Patients and their caregivers also bear the financial burden of readmissions and complex care.[4] Readmissions can lead to overall increased health care costs, including hospitalization, medications, diagnostic tests, and placement.[5] These costs place significant financial burden on patients, their families, and local health care systems (**Fig. 1**).

In many situations, patients may not have an adequate support system. Irreversible damage to the brain in addition to progressive hepatic decompensation and worsening neuropsychiatric functions can make it increasingly difficult to manage the disease alone.[6] For instance, patients may experience depression, anxiety, and social isolation, which can affect their ability to carry out daily activities and engage in meaningful relationships.[4] Even an easy call to the pharmacy for medication refills may become an

CYCLE OF HEPATIC ENCEPHALOPATHY READMISSION

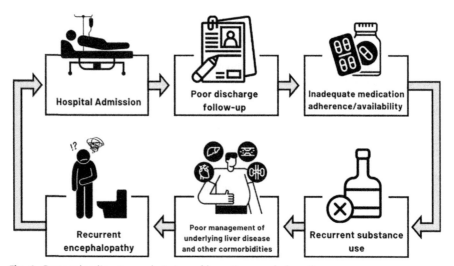

Fig. 1. Factors leading to readmission of hepatic encephalopathy.

impossible task for the patient. Given the detrimental impact of hepatic encephalopathy on mental, physical, and social functioning, identifying the specific areas of assistance required by the patient is essential in planning patient-specific modifications.

PRECIPITANTS OF HEPATIC ENCEPHALOPATHY

The presence of hepatic encephalopathy in several studies is strongly correlated with readmissions. In a study with 30-day readmission rates over 30%, hepatic encephalopathy was most strongly correlated with readmissions among underserved safety-net cirrhosis patients.[7] Similarly, one study reported a 30-day readmission rate of 23%, whereas a 90-day readmission rate in the setting of hepatic encephalopathy was approximately 38%.[8] Another study reported that a 1-year readmission rate for hepatic encephalopathy ranged from 31% to 43% which was significantly higher when compared with other portal hypertension complications such as ascites, variceal hemorrhage, hepatorenal syndrome, and hepatocellular carcinoma.[9]

The frequency of hospital admissions for hepatic encephalopathy can vary depending on the severity of liver disease. The recurrent nature relies on patient-specific strategies for identifying the precipitants of hepatic encephalopathy and appropriately treating the chronic illness. The most common precipitants for hepatic encephalopathy hospitalizations include polypharmacy (as well as medication adherence and acquisition), infections, gastrointestinal bleeding, constipation, dehydration, acute kidney injury, electrolyte abnormalities, inadequate management of comorbid conditions, alcohol consumption, and portosystemic shunts.[1,6,10] Several studies have emphasized these precipitating factors as common occurrences in hospital readmissions for hepatic encephalopathy. Identifying precipitating factors and treating the underlying etiology are critical before moving toward treatment specific for hepatic encephalopathy.

CYCLE OF HEPATIC ENCEPHALOPATHY READMISSIONS

The factors leading to readmission for hepatic encephalopathy are complex, warranting a multidisciplinary approach. For many, poor medication adherence and difficulties with medication acquisition may be the beginning of this vicious cycle. Inadequate discharge planning along with disjointed communication among health care providers can create significant gaps in care.[9,11] Patients without caregiver support are placed in unfavorable positions with limited access to help. Furthermore, the existing comorbidities in addition to the complications of recurrent hepatic encephalopathy further debilitate the patient. The multidisciplinary discharge strategies are vital in attacking these precipitating factors.

Common factors leading to readmission for hepatic encephalopathy include[5,7–9,11] (see **Fig. 1**):

- Inadequate medication acquisition and adherence to medications:
  - High costs or arduous prior authorization processes of obtaining rifaximin may be an insurmountable barrier for patients. These gaps lead to delay in the patient receiving outpatient medications for hepatic encephalopathy due to either insurance or provider issues that subsequently results in hospital readmission before the patient even starting outpatient treatment.
  - Patients with hepatic encephalopathy frequently need to take multiple medications, including lactulose and rifaximin. For example, lactulose is not tolerated by many patients due to its gastrointestinal side effects. Poor adherence to these medications increases the risk of decompensation and readmission.

- o The lack of education on medication side effects and drug interactions can negatively impact proper management of hepatic encephalopathy in the outpatient setting.
- Inadequate discharge planning:
  - o Inadequate planning or follow-up care results in care gaps. Effective discharge planning is essential in the transition from inpatient to outpatient settings.
  - o Prioritizing medication acquisition, scheduled follow-up appointments, and education on the disease can have a significant impact on preventing readmissions for hepatic encephalopathy.
  - o Check lists for providers at the time of discharge can assist in closing the gap in care. Involving the patient's support system and educating them with the patient can create a conducive environment for improvement.
- Inadequate post-discharge monitoring of precipitants:
  - o Awareness of precipitating factors and adequate preparation to address the various complications can help patients and their support system make decisions in times of uncertainty.
  - o The use of a self-care checklist should reinforce how to recognize signs of decompensation and close communication with the primary care provider during the post-discharge setting can address any concerns or changes in the patient's cognitive or functional status.
  - o Guidance from nutritionists, physical therapists, and social workers, for example, can reinforce lifestyle modifications through dietary changes, physical exercise, and avoidance of alcohol and other substance use.
- Inadequate post-discharge management of underlying liver disease and comorbidities:
  - o Liver disease can contribute to the development and exacerbation of hepatic encephalopathy. Inadequate management of complications of portal hypertension such as ascites and variceal bleeding can increase the risk of decompensation.
  - o Management of comorbidities such as renal disease, diabetes, and obesity should be controlled and followed closely with the patient's primary care team.
- Disjointed communication:
  - o Synchronous communication among health care providers can create a successful foundation to prevent a patient's clinical decline. Vital members of the health care team include nurses, pharmacists, social workers, nutritionists, physical therapists, hepatologists/gastroenterologists, and/or primary care providers.

APPROACH TO: ACQUISITION AND ADHERENCE OF MEDICATIONS

Preventing readmission for hepatic encephalopathy is complex and labor intensive, yet it is achievable. As readmission for hepatic encephalopathy has emerged as a significant issue for patients living with advanced liver disease, strategies need to be developed, implemented, and assessed to reduce the number of readmissions.[7] These strategies need to ensure patients can receive treatments for hepatic encephalopathy, that is, lactulose and rifaximin, in a timely and continuous manner.

The current treatment options for hepatic encephalopathy are the oral medications lactulose and rifaximin (**Fig. 2**). The use of lactulose in reducing hospital readmissions for hepatic encephalopathy is well-described in the literature. Lactulose is a liquid osmotic laxative, pulling water into the bowel leading to multiple bowel movements throughout the day. Lactulose is a nonabsorbable disaccharide metabolized and fermented by colonic bacteria, which has a cathartic effect leading to a decrease in blood

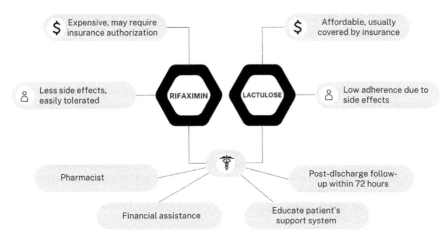

Fig. 2. Factors related to hepatic encephalopathy treatment: rifaximin versus lactulose.

ammonia concentration and increased fecal nitrogen excretion with up to a fourfold increase in stool volume.[12-14] At home, patients are recommended to take 15 to 30 mL of lactulose, two to four times a day to reach at least two semisoft stools per day. Owing to the lactulose mechanism of action, patients experience significant gastrointestinal side effects such as diarrhea, abdominal cramps, and bloating.[12,15] Therefore, patient tolerance and adherence to lactulose is generally low. Overuse of lactulose can also lead to dehydration, hypernatremia, and anal skin irritation.[14,16] The difficulty for patients to remain compliant to lactulose leads to recurrent hepatic encephalopathy and readmission.

Rifaximin, a broad-spectrum semisynthetic oral antibiotic, has transformed the patient experience in the treatment of hepatic encephalopathy. With minimal drug–drug interactions, adverse effects, and the lack of dose adjustments required due to concomitant medical conditions, rifaximin has become the mainstay of therapy to reduce the risk of hepatic encephalopathy.[16,17] At home, patients are recommended to take one rifaximin 550 mg tablet, twice a day. Rifaximin use, as compared with the use of lactulose, has been shown to significantly reduce the mean number of hospitalizations and mean days of hospitalizations for hepatic encephalopathy[18] In another study, the combination of rifaximin and lactulose described a significantly lower risk (78%) of breakthrough hepatic encephalopathy when compared with 54% patients in the placebo group.[19] Thus, the use of rifaximin and the combination of rifaximin and lactulose are strong predictors to reduce recurrence of hepatic encephalopathy and hospital readmissions. Rifaximin, with or without lactulose, has been shown to decrease hospital readmissions for recurrent hepatic encephalopathy.[20] On hospital discharge, patients receiving rifaximin during the hospital stay are often prescribed to continue this in the outpatient setting.

Several challenges exist for patients prescribed rifaximin. Patients often return to the hospital due to medication-related issues, but the cause requires further investigation. Decline in memory causes patients to simply forget to take their medications and may also affect the patient's ability to call the pharmacy for medication refills. In severe cases, picking up and dialing a phone number may be a challenge for a patient. Once an easy daily task, the simple act of dialing a telephone can become an impossible chore. Other obstacles include the price of medication, the prior authorization process required by many insurance carriers, and delays in follow-up with medical providers.[5]

A delay of 7 days in obtaining the rifaximin is associated with recurrent hepatic encephalopathy and hospital readmission.[21]

Ideally, during the patient's hospital stay, the multidisciplinary team should develop a care plan to ensure patients receive enough supply of rifaximin to bridge the gap between discharge and medical follow-up. Unfortunately, most of the admitted hepatic encephalopathy patients do not receive proper therapeutic management after discharge. An analysis of medical and hospital claims by Neff and colleagues reported that greater than 60% of patients who had more than one episode of hepatic encephalopathy did not receive ongoing treatments to reduce the risk of hepatic encephalopathy recurrence on hospital discharge to the outpatient setting.[22] To expedite and ensure patients will have access to rifaximin at home, the multidisciplinary team should send prescriptions to the patient's home pharmacy and if necessary, submit the prior authorization during the hospital stay (**Fig. 3**). The cost of copay should also be assessed, as copays may range from $0 to thousands of dollars each month.

APPROACH TO DISCHARGE PLANNING

The preventable nature of hepatic encephalopathy is key to creating optimal strategies, especially in the discharge and post-discharge settings. In a retrospective study, Saab and colleagues found hepatic encephalopathy to be both a common and preventable cause of readmission within 1 month of discharge in patients with decompensated cirrhosis.[1]

Most of the patients will improve significantly while in the hospital to the point where they can be discharged. Treatment for the primary diagnosis is important but creating a care plan to prevent the readmission is vital. Early planning for patient discharge will allow the multidisciplinary team time to plan and support the patient accordingly.

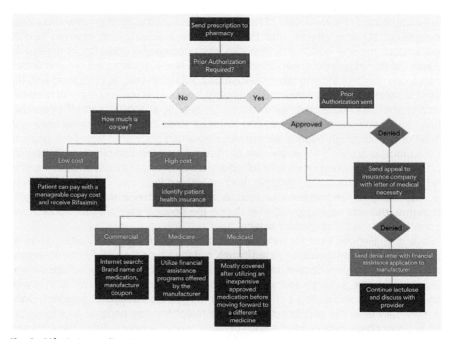

Fig. 3. Rifaximin medication acquisition process map.

Patient-centered plans can ensure a smooth transition from the hospital to the community setting (**Fig. 4**).

When a patient is ready for hospital discharge, health care providers typically assess their functional status, cognitive ability, and other social factors that may impact their ability to manage their condition in the outpatient setting. This assessment should involve a multidisciplinary team, including physicians, nurses, pharmacists, nutritionists, social workers, physical therapist, and other health care professionals. A comprehensive checklist for the health care team preparing for discharge can ensure a complete assessment of the patients' needs (**Box 1**).

In general, discharge planning for patients with hepatic encephalopathy involves addressing the following issues.

- *Medication management:* Patients must be given clear instructions on how and when to take their medications, including dosage, frequency, and potential side effects. They should receive education on how to manage any potential side effects. The discharge planning team needs to ensure patients are able to fill prescriptions for lactulose and/or rifaximin either at the hospital pharmacy on discharge or at a local pharmacy on the day of discharge. This means that discharge planning teams need to either complete the prior authorization process before discharge or provide the patient with at least a 7-day supply of medication, whereas the prior authorization process proceeds (see **Fig. 3**). If these criteria cannot be met, discharge is discouraged until the team and patient is secure in being able to obtain the medication for outpatient use.
- *Cognitive and functional assessment:* Patients should be assessed for any cognitive or functional deficits related to hepatic encephalopathy, such as difficulty with memory, attention, or motor function. They may receive recommendations

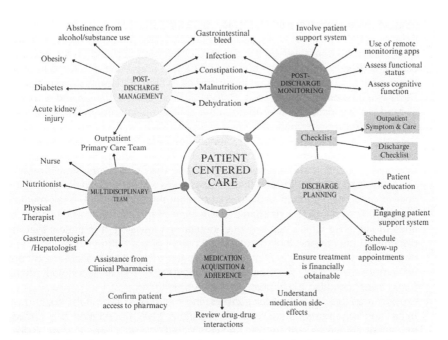

Fig. 4. Multidisciplinary approach to patient-centered care for hepatic encephalopathy.

Box 1
Preparing for discharge: health care team checklist for patients with hepatic encephalopathy

- What is the patient's functional and cognitive status at the time of discharge? Are physical therapists, nutritionists, and social workers involved in care?
- Are the patient's family or caregivers involved and available for the patient? If so, have they seen any changes in the patient's functional or cognitive status when compared with baseline?
- Does the patient and/or caregivers know the precipitants (infection, bleeding, volume depletion, and so forth) of hepatic encephalopathy?
- Can the patient and/or caregivers recognize the signs of recurrence (confusion, tremors, delirium, and so forth)? If so, do they know when and how to reach out to the providers?
- Does the patient and/or caregivers know signs or symptoms that are commonly mistaken for hepatic encephalopathy and favor a different medical condition?
- If the patient has a prior history of alcohol use, did the patient get any post-discharge rehabilitation or resources to help with abstinence?
- Does the patient have a scheduled appointment for follow-up with their primary care physician and/or specialist?
- Does the patient have medications ready for their hepatic encephalopathy at the time of discharge with instructions in hand?
- Did we provide the patient with a helpline for patients and their caregivers?

---

for behavioral modifications or exercises and potential rehabilitation or other therapies to help improve their functional status.

- *Follow-up appointments:* Patients should be scheduled for follow-up appointments with their health care provider to monitor their condition and adjust their treatments as needed in a timely fashion, generally within 3 to 5 days of discharge. If the outpatient provider is not part of in-hospital care team, the outpatient provider should be contacted by the discharge team and updated on the patient's current condition and discharge plan. The patient may also be referred to other health care providers or community resources to help manage their condition.
- *Review of medication interactions:* Before discharge, a discussion and review of all medications including over-the-counter and complementary/alternative therapies should be performed with the patient and their health care support team. Patients at risk of alcohol use and potential dependency on sedative treatments may benefit from referral to an inpatient or outpatient rehabilitation program.
- *Caregiver education and support:* Patients and their caregivers should receive education and support to help them manage the patient's condition, including how to recognize signs of hepatic encephalopathy and when to seek medical attention. They should be instructed about early intervention with additional dosages of lactulose which can prevent hospital readmission. It is critical that the discharged patient and their caregiver be aware of the outpatient provider and have the provider's office 24/7 contact information. Providing available resources for remote monitoring, such as patient checklists or mobile technology monitoring apps, can also aid in post-discharge monitoring.
- *Provide available resources for patients and caregivers:* Hospitals, health systems, and organizations such as the American Liver Foundation can provide outpatient resources and support services to patients with hepatic encephalopathy and their families, friends, and caregivers. Information regarding these

services should be given to the patient and their caregivers by the care team on hospital discharge.

APPROACH TO POST-DISCHARGE MONITORING OF PRECIPITANTS AND MANAGEMENT OF COMORBIDITIES

There are several common precipitants that increase the risk of developing hepatic encephalopathy (**Table 1**). On hospital discharge, it is important to make patients aware of the signs and symptoms of these precipitating factors. Patients should receive an at-home self-help checklist to guide them with symptom management. An example is shown in **Table 2**. Informed patients can appropriately address these factors in a timely manner before they develop hepatic encephalopathy. This may decrease the recurrence rate of hepatic encephalopathy and lower readmission rates.

- *Cognitive and functional assessment:* Patients should be monitored for any cognitive or functional changes such as difficulty with memory, attention, or motor function. Participation with a physical therapist at home or in a rehabilitation facility can help monitor progress. If a patient is independent at home, maintaining a record of any new changes to the cognitive or physical status must be kept. The use of remote monitoring systems through mobile technology or computer applications are available. However, a simple patient diary is also beneficial.
- *Gastrointestinal bleeding:* Hemorrhage is a common precipitating factor leading to hepatic encephalopathy. In patients with variceal hemorrhage, ensuring a treatment and maintenance plan such as the use of nonselective beta-blockers and/or gastric variceal band ligation may prevent recurrent variceal bleeding.[6]
- *Constipation:* Infrequent bowel movements is a frequent predisposing factor to the development of hepatic encephalopathy, presumably secondary to increased ammonia absorption from the gut due to slow transit time.[23] Ensuring a care plan to prevent the development of constipation in recently hospitalized patients, such as the increased use of fiber or laxatives to promote adequate bowel movements, can prevent recurrent hepatic encephalopathy. Adherence to lactulose also aids in preventing recurrent hepatic encephalopathy and hospital readmission.
- *Infections,* in particular, spontaneous bacterial peritonitis, cellulitis, urinary tract infection, and pneumonia can all precipitate hepatic encephalopathy. On discharge, antibiotics should be continued as recommended. To prevent recurrent spontaneous bacterial peritonitis, prophylactic antibiotic should be continued. In the outpatient setting, vigilance in recognizing symptoms of infections and timely treatment is important in preventing recurrent hepatic encephalopathy.
- *Dehydration* secondary to volume depletion and *electrolyte imbalances*, such as hyponatremia and hypokalemia, can lead to recurrent hepatic encephalopathy by disrupting the cellular membrane potentials.[10] Patients should avoid volume depletion caused by over diuresis through appropriate medication management and be encouraged to maintain adequate oral hydration. Maintaining adequate hydration and electrolyte management in the outpatient setting can prevent hospital readmission for hepatic encephalopathy.
- Patients with cirrhosis commonly present with nutritional deficiencies. Malnutrition, particularly of protein and vitamins, can increase the risk of hepatic encephalopathy by affecting liver function and brain metabolism. Protein restriction is associated with increased mortality in these patients; therefore, patients with a history of hepatic encephalopathy should not be placed on a restricted protein diet.[24]
- A post-discharge, outpatient management of concomitant medical conditions is imperative to prevent recurrent hepatic encephalopathy and hospital

Table 1
Precipitants of hepatic encephalopathy

Precipitating Factors	Description	Solution
Gastrointestinal bleeding	Common with variceal hemorrhage and peptic ulcer disease	Nonselective beta-blockers, band ligation, antacid therapies
Constipation	Presumed secondary to increased ammonia absorption in setting of slow gut transit time.	Increase fiber intake and utilization of laxatives including lactulose
Infections	Poor immunity, high risk of infection	Hygiene, maintain distance from others with known infection, and improve frailty scores
Electrolyte imbalance and Dehydration	Can lead to disruption of cellular membrane	Monitoring electrolyte and hydration
Malnutrition	Deficiency in protein and vitamins	Nutrition education, avoid protein restrictive diet
Concomitant medical condition	Comorbid conditions such as diabetes, heart disease, and renal disease	Appropriate outpatient management of concomitant medical conditions with primary care team.
Contraindicated medication and/or substance use	Use of sedatives, opioids, benzodiazepines, illicit drugs	Education and review of medication intake; use of available clinical pharmacist

Table 2
Outpatient symptom and care check list

Questions to Ask Oneself	Why Is This Question Important to Me	How Can I Help Myself?	When Should I Call My Doctor?
Am I throwing up blood (coffee ground)? Are my bowel movements black?	*Gastrointestinal bleeding:* It can be life-threatening. This is commonly seen in variceal bleeding or peptic ulcer disease.	To prevent GI bleeding, you can take medications as prescribed by your doctor including: nonselective beta blockers, undergo band ligation, and/or antiacids.	You should call your doctor immediately.
Did I have enough bowel movements today?	*Constipation:* Bowel movements prevent buildup of toxin that can worsen my mental functions.	Monitor your daily bowel movement goal.	If you are constipated, in addition to lactulose, ask your doctor what else you can do.
Did I drink enough water today? Am I urinating enough?	*Dehydration/volume depletion:* Not drinking enough water can lead to dehydration and increase the risk of confusion.	Make sure to drink enough water.	When you feel symptomatic, call the doctor.
I am getting more confused?	*Confusion:* is a sign of encephalopathy.	Increase the amount and frequency of lactulose to treat your symptoms.	If there is no improvement with dose modulation, call your doctor.
Do I have fever, chills, abdominal pain, and/or feel unwell?	*Fever and chills:* can be signs of infection.	Drink fluids, take acetaminophen, and monitor your symptoms.	If no improvement, call your doctor immediately.
Do I live alone and notice changes in my mental status?	*Changes in mental status:* in the setting of being alone can be dangerous.	Call your support system and make them aware of your mental status changes.	Call your doctor immediately.

readmission. Medical conditions, such as diabetes, heart disease especially heart failure, pulmonary disease, and chronic kidney disease, can increase the risk of hepatic encephalopathy by affecting liver function and the metabolic processes in the body. Close follow-up with primary care physician and specialists should not be delayed.

- The use of certain medications, in particular sedatives, opioids, benzodiazepines, and antidepressants, can increase the risk of hepatic encephalopathy by affecting brain function and reducing the ability of the liver to metabolize toxins. Proton-pump inhibitors are known to be a predictor of the development of hepatic encephalopathy.[25] Clinicians should discontinue proton-pump inhibitors when clinically appropriate, given the increased risk of hepatic encephalopathy. The use of alcohol or illicit drugs can also increase the risk of recurrent hepatic encephalopathy and hospital readmission.

APPROACH TO MULTIDISCIPLINARY CARE

A multidisciplinary team approach is the key to managing the complexity of hepatic encephalopathy that can be debilitating for the patient, caregiver, family, and hospital system. On discharge, a nutritionist and physical therapist can assist with proper nutrition, hydration, and daily exercises to train the patient to adapt back into society. It is vital to have, if possible, a clinical pharmacist on the care team to answer questions and review potential drug–drug interactions that can lead to recurrent hepatic encephalopathy. A well-coordinated team can prevent hospital readmission. Although obvious, it is important to state that the prevention of readmission for hepatic encephalopathy improves overall patient quality of life. These efforts are cost-saving to medical centers and the overall health care system. The use of experts such as pharmacists, social workers, nutritionists, and physical therapists on these care teams are cost-effective and improve patient and provider quality of life and therefore should help decrease the recurrence rate of hepatic encephalopathy and decrease hospital readmissions for hepatic encephalopathy.

APPROACH TO THE READMITTED PATIENT: PERSPECTIVE FOR THE HEALTH CARE WORKER

The unpredictable nature of hepatic encephalopathy makes it a challenging diagnosis. Patients with hepatic encephalopathy have significant impairments in their cognitive, physical, and social functioning. During the evaluation of a patient who is readmitted for recurrent encephalopathy, it is essential to see the patient as *whole*. It is critical to have curiosity and interest in the patient's life and daily functions before their admission. The reason(s) for readmission may be multifactorial. Therefore, it is important to understand that the primary cause of patient's hospital admission may not be so apparent. Nonadherence to medication is different from not being able to afford the medication. Hepatic encephalopathy is a condition that declines a patient's ability to carry out their daily tasks. Recurrence of delirium may be from the lack of outpatient follow-up or support to maneuver daily activities. Every patient presents on a spectrum; the level of change in daily functions can be gradual for some and drastic for others. Patient's self-perception can be deceiving; therefore, engaging family, friends, and caregivers is essential to fully comprehend the patient's outpatient situation. The unity of a patient, their support system, and a multidisciplinary health care team can have a significant impact in preventing readmission in hepatic encephalopathy moving forward.

SUMMARY

Readmission rates for patients with hepatic encephalopathy are significantly higher than those of other complications of advanced liver disease. This high recurrence rate and subsequent readmission rate decreases patient quality of life. Many of these readmissions for hepatic encephalopathy are preventable. Most patients with the discharge diagnosis of hepatic encephalopathy do not receive appropriate ongoing outpatient treatments for this condition which results in a high early readmission rate. Multidisciplinary discharge planning teams must address all the transition issues from inpatient to outpatient before discharge if readmission rates due to hepatic encephalopathy are to be reduced. After discharge, patients require close follow up and management through in person office visits and enhanced telephone management. Prevention of hospital readmission due to hepatic encephalopathy requires close collaboration between healthcare providers, patients, and caregivers to optimize the patient's overall health and well-being.

DISCLOSURE

The authors of this research paper declare that they have no financial, personal, or professional interest that could be perceived as influencing the research findings or conclusions presented in this article. There are no conflicts of interest, affiliations, or funding sources to disclose.

REFERENCES

1. Saab S. Evaluation of the impact of rehospitalization in the management of hepatic encephalopathy. Int J Gen Med 2015;8:165–73.

2. Atluri DK, Prakash R, Mullen KD. Pathogenesis, diagnosis, and treatment of hepatic encephalopathy. J Clin Exp Hepatol 2011;1(2):77–86.

3. Sotil EU, Gottstein J, Ayala E, et al. Impact of preoperative overt hepatic encephalopathy on neurocognitive function after liver transplantation. Liver Transpl 2009; 15(2):184–92.

4. Agrawal S, Umapathy S, Dhiman RK. Minimal hepatic encephalopathy impairs quality of life. J Clin Exp Hepatol 2015;5(Suppl 1):S42–8.

5. Flamm SL, Bajaj JS, Saab S, et al. The role of the hospitalist in the continuum of care for patients with hepatic encephalopathy: treatment of inpatient episodes and preventing outpatient recurrence and readmissions. Journal of Hospital Management and Health Policy 2020;4.

6. Louissaint J, Deutsch-Link S, Tapper EB. Changing Epidemiology of cirrhosis and hepatic encephalopathy. Clin Gastroenterol Hepatol 2022;20(8S):S1–8.

7. Sood KT, Wong RJ. Hepatic encephalopathy is a strong predictor of early hospital readmission among cirrhosis patients. J Clin Exp Hepatol 2019;9(4):484–90.

8. Bajaj JS, Reddy KR, Tandon P, et al. The 3-month readmission rate remains unacceptably high in a large North American cohort of patients with cirrhosis. Hepatology 2016;64(1):200–8.

9. Tapper EB, Halbert B, Mellinger J. Rates of and reasons for hospital readmissions in patients with cirrhosis: a Multistate Population-based cohort study. Clin Gastroenterol Hepatol 2016;14(8):1181–8.e2.

10. Shaw J, Beyers L, Bajaj JS. Inadequate practices for hepatic encephalopathy management in the inpatient setting. J Hosp Med 2022;17(Suppl 1):S8–16.

11. Rosenstengle C, Kripalani S, Rahimi RS. Hepatic encephalopathy and strategies to prevent readmission from inadequate transitions of care. J Hosp Med 2022; 17(Suppl 1):S17–23.

12. Conn HO, Leevy CM, Vlahcevic ZR, et al. Comparison of lactulose and neomycin in the treatment of chronic portal-systemic encephalopathy. A double blind controlled trial. Gastroenterology 1977;72(4 Pt 1):573–83.

13. Morgan MY. Current state of knowledge of hepatic encephalopathy (part III): non-absorbable disaccharides. Metab Brain Dis 2016;31(6):1361–4.

14. Vilstrup H, Amodio P, Bajaj J, et al. Hepatic encephalopathy in chronic liver disease: 2014 Practice Guideline by the American association for the study of liver diseases and the European association for the study of the liver. Hepatology 2014;60(2):715–35.

15. Rahimi RS, Singal AG, Cuthbert JA, et al. Lactulose vs polyethylene glycol 3350–electrolyte solution for treatment of overt hepatic encephalopathy: the HELP randomized clinical trial. JAMA Intern Med 2014;174(11):1727–33.

16. Patidar KR, Bajaj JS. Covert and overt hepatic encephalopathy: diagnosis and management. Clin Gastroenterol Hepatol 2015;13(12):2048–61.

17. Sharma BC, Sharma P, Lunia MK, et al. A randomized, double-blind, controlled trial comparing rifaximin plus lactulose with lactulose alone in treatment of overt hepatic encephalopathy. Am J Gastroenterol 2013;108(9):1458–63.

18. Leevy CB, Phillips JA. Hospitalizations during the use of rifaximin versus lactulose for the treatment of hepatic encephalopathy. Dig Dis Sci 2007;52(3):737–41.

19. Bass NM, Mullen KD, Sanyal A, et al. Rifaximin treatment in hepatic encephalopathy. N Engl J Med 2010;362(12):1071–81.

20. Hudson M, Schuchmann M. Long-term management of hepatic encephalopathy with lactulose and/or rifaximin: a review of the evidence. Eur J Gastroenterol Hepatol 2019;31(4):434–50.

21. Stoll AM, Guido M, Pence A, et al. Lack of access to rifaximin upon hospital discharge is frequent and results in increased hospitalizations for hepatic encephalopathy. Ann Pharmacother 2023;57(2):133–40.

22. Neff GW, Frederick RT. Assessing treatment patterns in patients with overt hepatic encephalopathy. Hoboken (NJ): WILEY-BLACKWELL; 2012. p. 945A.

23. Sharma M, Anjum H, Bulathsinghala CP, et al. An Intriguing case of acute encephalopathy: Lesson Learned from a constipated man. Cureus 2020;12(1): e6678.

24. Bajaj JS. Review article: the modern management of hepatic encephalopathy. Aliment Pharmacol Ther 2010;31(5):537–47.

25. Bian J, Wang A, Lin J, et al. Association between proton pump inhibitors and hepatic encephalopathy: a meta-analysis. Medicine (Baltim) 2017;96(17):e6723.

Preventing Readmissions of Hepatic Encephalopathy

Strategies in the Acute Inpatient, Immediate Postdischarge, and Longitudinal Outpatient Setting

Emily Lin, MD[a], Devika Gandhi, MD[a],*, Michael Volk, MD, MSc[b]

KEYWORDS

- Decompensated cirrhosis • Hepatic encephalopathy • Hospital readmission
- Cirrhosis complications • Morbidity • Chronic liver disease • Hospitalization

KEY POINTS

- Hepatic encephalopathy (HE) is a strong predictor of early hospital readmission in patients with cirrhosis, early hospital readmission increases health care costs and is associated with worse survival.
- In the inpatient setting, strategies such as utilization of hepatology–hospitalist team comanagement, involvement of a multidisciplinary team, and utilization of electronic health record checklists can help prevent HE readmissions.
- In the immediate postdischarge setting, the implementation of a transitional care team who follows up with the patient and their caregivers can help prevent HE readmissions.
- In the longitudinal outpatient setting, pharmacy and medication-based interventions, community-based day programs, technological-based applications, and novel approaches such as titrating medication to Bristol Stool Scale or utilization of fecal microbiota transplant can be leveraged to help prevent HE readmissions.

INTRODUCTION

Hepatic encephalopathy (HE) is a strong predictor of early hospital readmission in patients with cirrhosis,[1,2] with a median readmission rate in published studies of 26% by 30 days after discharge.[1] Early hospital readmission increases health care costs and is associated with worse survival.[3] In fact, patients with cirrhosis have an estimated increased resource utilization at >$17 billion per year in the Medicare population in the United States.[2] Patients with cirrhosis experiencing early readmission also have

[a] Department of Gastroenterology, Loma Linda University, Loma Linda, CA, USA; [b] Department of Medicine, Baylor Scott and White, Central Texas Region, Temple, TX, USA
* Corresponding author. 11234 Anderson Street, Loma Linda, CA 92354.
E-mail address: devikagandhi@llu.edu

Clin Liver Dis 28 (2024) 359–367
https://doi.org/10.1016/j.cld.2024.01.010
1089-3261/24/© 2024 Elsevier Inc. All rights reserved.
liver.theclinics.com

greater 90 day, 1 year, and overall mortality.[3] Fortunately, studies have shown these readmissions are partially preventable. Herein we provide an overview of strategies to prevent hospital readmissions in patients with HE, divided into 3 contexts: (a) acute inpatient, (b) immediate postdischarge, and (c) longitudinal outpatient setting (**Fig. 1**).

STRATEGIES
Strategies in the Acute Inpatient Setting

Comanagement between specialty teams and internists
One approach for preventing HE readmissions involves increased comanagement between hepatologists and internists when caring for patients with cirrhosis in the inpatient setting. By more fully integrating the expertise of hepatologist consultants, this intervention can improve adherence to the most current evidence-based practices and guidelines for treating patients with cirrhosis. In one study by Desai and colleagues, the researchers demonstrated the effectiveness of a comanagement strategy in which patients with cirrhosis admitted for spontaneous bacterial peritonitis (SBP) were concentrated to a single hospital unit which allowed for daily evaluation by both the primary hospitalist and consulting hepatology team and more frequent multidisciplinary discussions between both teams.[4] This intervention ultimately led to significantly better management of SBP, including a significant increase in timely paracentesis and appropriate use of albumin infusions. Although that study focused specifically on outcomes in patients with SBP, restructuring the inpatient service framework to allow for more dedicated guidance from hepatology consultants also has the potential to improve adherence to standard practice guidelines when managing patients with HE.

Involvement of ancillary staff and nonphysician team members
An increasing number of nonphysician providers and ancillary staff are taking on crucial roles in the management of patients with cirrhosis. A multidisciplinary team of health care personnel including advanced practice providers (APP), pharmacists, and dieticians, helps ensure better delivery of care for hospitalized patients with

Strategies to Prevent Hepatic Encephalopathy Readmissions

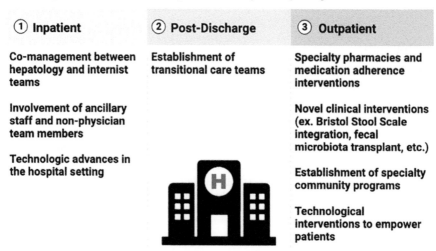

① Inpatient	② Post-Discharge	③ Outpatient
Co-management between hepatology and internist teams	Establishment of transitional care teams	Specialty pharmacies and medication adherence interventions
Involvement of ancillary staff and non-physician team members		Novel clinical interventions (ex. Bristol Stool Scale integration, fecal microbiota transplant, etc.)
Technologic advances in the hospital setting		Establishment of specialty community programs
		Technological interventions to empower patients

Fig. 1. Strategies to prevent hepatic encephalopathy readmissions.

cirrhosis by allowing physicians to focus on other matters such as transplant listing and leveraging their respective expertise. In one study by Tapper and colleagues that compared outcomes in patients with HE subdivided into groups with and without APP comanagement, the comanaged group had a significantly increased rate of rifaximin compliance as well as decreased 30 day readmission rates.[5] Inpatient pharmacists are another group that play an integral role in improving patient education in the hospital setting which in turn leads to favorable health care outcomes.[6–9] Though there are no recent studies that have examined pharmacist-led interventions specifically in patients with cirrhosis, multiple studies have demonstrated that patients who received pharmacist-led medication education had a greater than 10% decreased incidence of readmissions in the 12 months following hospitalization compared with patients who did not receive pharmacist-directed education.[8,10] Finally, early involvement of dieticians for hospitalized patients with cirrhosis has been associated with favorable patient outcomes. Sarcopenia and myosteatosis are highly prevalent in patients with cirrhosis and have been shown to be associated with overt HE as loss of muscle mass decreases the ability of skeletal muscle to effectively clear ammonia from the body.[11,12] In one notable study by Shaw and colleagues, the researchers demonstrated that involving dieticians early in the hospitalization course to help address nutritional deficiencies in patients with cirrhosis has been associated with both reduced length of stay and 90 day readmissions.[6] Taken together, these studies highlight how involving nonphysician team members allows for comprehensive patient care to patients with cirrhosis in the hospital setting, which is crucial for preventing future unnecessary hospitalizations.

Technological advances in the hospital setting

The utilization of new technologic advances and automated systems in hospitals is an effective technique to ensure standardized care for patients with cirrhosis and prevent readmissions due to HE. In one study involving patients with cirrhosis hospitalized for encephalopathy, Tapper and colleagues demonstrated that the implementing checklists in the electronic ordering system that allowed providers to order medications like lactulose and rifaximin by default led to a 38% lower risk for HE readmission as well as decreased length of stay.[13] In another prospective study by Louissaint and colleagues, the researchers found that implementing an interruptive electronic medical record alert to remind providers to start rifaximin in patients with HE already on lactulose led to increased rifaximin utilization, particularly on nongastroenterology services, which in turn led to lower readmission rates.[14] Overall, integration of automated checklists and alerts in the electronic medical system has potential to improve provider adherence to current best practices for treating patients with cirrhosis and potentially avoid preventable readmissions due to HE.

Strategies in the Immediate Postdischarge Setting

Establishment of transitional care teams

The creation of transitional care teams whose goal is to implement strategies that safely transit patients from the inpatient to outpatient setting has recently emerged as an area for potentially improving patient outcomes and preventing hospital readmissions. In one single-center study, Kripalani and colleagues showed that utilizing care coordinator nurses who conducted early telephone follow up and provided postdischarge education to patients and caregivers following discharge led to significantly reduced readmissions within 30 and 90 days compared with instances where only the physician provided education of when no designated discharge call was made.[15] Of note, there are several pilot studies to date that have demonstrated the utilization of transitional care teams specifically in the HE patient population. These studies showed that readmissions were significantly reduced in patients who received brief targeted outpatient education on HE treatment plans, early postdischarge telephone call within 72 hours, and had close follow up with transitional care providers compared with patients who did not receive these interventions.[16,17] These findings were further corroborated by Yoder and colleagues who revealed that patients who attended a postdischarge liver clinic facilitated by transitional care multidisciplinary team (involving physician assistants, nursing, social work, nutrition, and pharmacy) had a significant decrease in 30 day readmissions compared with nonattendees (12% vs 22%, respectively).[18] Altogether, these studies underscore the advantages of having a specialized transitional care team during the immediate postdischarge period to help mitigate the risk of readmissions and other complications related to cirrhosis.

Strategies in the Longitudinal Outpatient Setting

Specialty pharmacies and medication adherence interventions
The current standard-of-care treatment of HE includes lactulose, with the addition of rifaximin for patients who fail lactulose monotherapy.[19,20] Numerous studies have demonstrated the effectiveness of these medications in decreasing risk of breakthrough episodes of overt HE and lowering 30 day readmission rates from both all-causes and cirrhosis-related processes.[20–22] Unfortunately, medication nonadherence is a major precipitant of HE, and survey data have demonstrated that a major driver of poor medication adherence is high medication costs.[8] One study by Bajaj and colleagues showed that as much as 46% of patients were nonadherent with lactulose after an initial episode of HE due to high medication costs, and that 82.0% of the nonadherent patients failed to fill their prescription regularly.[23] Prior studies also reveal that 3 in 10 patients have problems affording HE therapy, and that out-of-pocket copay for rifaximin can range anywhere from $200 to more than $1000 per month for patients with inadequate insurance.[22,24,25] One proposed strategy to address this issue is raising patient and clinician awareness of specialty pharmacies who can assist with obtaining insurance approvals and accessing otherwise costly prescription medications such as rifaximin.[24] In one meta-analysis by Kini and colleagues, researchers also showed that consulting clinical pharmacists for disease comanagement, which involved providing patient education, enhancing disease monitoring via more frequent telephone or in-person follow up visits, and issuing refill reminders, also led to a 15% increase in medication adherence.[26] Though not specifically studied in the population with cirrhosis, other interventions that have been shown to improve medication adherence include the use of medication packaging interventions such as pill-boxes or blister packaging as well as the use of combination pills to reduce daily pill burden. Separate meta-analysis studies have demonstrated that these interventions can increase medication compliance by approximately 10%.[26,27] Although the feasibility of implementing these interventions need to be evaluated in the population with cirrhosis, integrating these practices into the management of patients with HE could play an integral role in averting unnecessary rehospitalizations and high health care costs.

Novel clinical practices to personalize hepatic encephalopathy management
For patients with cirrhosis being treated with lactulose, conventional thinking among health care practitioners was that achieving a certain number of bowel movements while on lactulose therapy implied treatment efficacy.[28] However, a significant proportion of patients may be vulnerable to multiple adverse effects associated with overtitrating of their medication dosages, such as dehydration, electrolyte derangements,

and gastrointestinal symptoms.[29] This in turn can lead to poor medication adherence and subsequent unnecessary hospitalizations, prompting the need for tools other than bowel movement frequency to help adjust medication in the outpatient setting. One proposed tool is the Bristol stool scale (BSS), a patient-reported characterization on stool consistency ranging from 1 through 7 that has been historically validated in conditions such as Clostridioides difficile infections.[30,31] More recently, BSS has been suggested as a new adjunctive marker of treatment response in patients undergoing lactulose therapy.[32,33] In one notable study that compared outcomes in patients in whom only stool frequency was used to determine management versus those in whom both stool frequency and BSS were considered, the researchers revealed a lower 6 month total or HE-related admission rate associated with the BSS group.[33] The study's findings suggest that BSS can serve as a valuable tool for evaluating treatment response in patients on lactulose treatment, which in turn can help circumvent the potential risks and complications associated with dose escalation based solely on bowel movement frequency.[33,34] Thus, incorporating tools like BSS into the management of patients with cirrhosis in the outpatient setting can help personalize therapy plans to the individual patient to improve medication compliance, and ultimately potentially lower the risk of HE-related readmissions.

Another strategy that has recently emerged for preventing HE events in patients with cirrhosis is the introduction of fecal microbiota transplant (FMT). The pathophysiology behind recurrent HE is linked with microbial dysbiosis and a reduction of healthy gut flora which eventually leads to cognitive impairment and systemic inflammation.[35,36] FMT is a procedure that directly targets the gastrointestinal microbial composition of patients with HE by administering healthy donor fecal matter into the gastrointestinal tract, which is particularly useful in patients not responding to the standard of care (SOC) regimen of lactulose and rifaximin.[37] In one randomized clinical trial by Bajaj and colleagues, 20 patients with recurrent HE receiving SOC were randomly assigned to either receive FMT treatment or not.[37] The researchers found that patients who received FMT in addition to SOC had significantly lower incidence of HE events at 5 months postrandomization compared with the SOC group (0 vs 6, respectively), as well as significant improvements in HE-related cognitive test scores compared with patients receiving lactulose and rifaximin alone. Although the efficacy of FMT in patients with cirrhosis still needs to be validated in larger, prospective studies, it is a promising strategy for treating difficult, refractory HE cases which can help mitigate the risk of rehospitalization.

Establishment of specialty community programs

Specialized community-based outpatient programs have also shown great potential in managing patients with cirrhosis and reducing unnecessary readmissions related to HE. One such program is the hepatology day unit hospital which permits access to health care services that otherwise would have been done in an inpatient hospital setting. Clinicians are able to order rapid laboratory and radiological testing, conduct psychometric evaluations for the diagnosis of HE, and even perform procedures like outpatient paracentesis and endoscopies depending on the needs of the patient.[38–40] The benefits of this outpatient program are highlighted in one study by Morando and colleagues in which patients admitted for decompensated cirrhosis were randomized into 2 groups, one of which received close follow up in a hepatology day unit hospital following discharge while the other did not. The investigators found that patients with close follow up in the hepatology day unit hospital had decreased relative risk of 30 day readmission compared with those in the standard outpatient group (11.3% vs 29.5%), as well as lower 1-year mortality (23.1% vs 45.7%) and reduced overall cost.[38] Ultimately, the emergence of community-based programs such as the hepatology day unit hospital represents a new model of specialized health care services that can significantly enhance patients' access to health care in the outpatient setting and thus decrease the need for hospitalizations.

Technological interventions to empower patients

Two major factors contribute to frequent readmissions in cirrhotic patients with HE: (1) failure to address common precipitants of HE such as medication nonadherence and (2) failure to prevent the condition from progressing to overt encephalopathy in a timely manner. The integration of automated digital technologies including text messaging and smartphone applications into patient care has been shown to be a promising strategy to tackle these issues.[41] In one study by Thakkar and colleagues, investigators found that daily text messages reminding patients to take their medications increased the odds of medication adherence by almost double compared with patients who did no text messaging.[42] The use of text messaging reminders in patient care has also been studied specifically in the cirrhosis patient population. In one trial study involving 40 patients with HE who were followed for 30 days postdischarge, Ganapathy and colleagues introduced the idea of a smartphone application known as "Patient Buddy" which allowed patients and caregivers to record daily medication adherence, track sodium intake and body weight, and conduct weekly cognitive and fall risk assessments at home.[43] If there were critical values or missing entries of critical medications, this automatically alerted the monitoring clinical team and prompted communication to the patient. Of note, the researchers demonstrated that 8 potential HE-related hospitalizations were prevented through app-generated alerts that encouraged patients to seek early outpatient interventions within 24 hours.

New advances in technology also have the potential to educate patients on symptom monitoring at home and help them recognize progression in their disease. This in turn allows for timely interventions to be initiated once covert or minimally overt HE is recognized. In one study by Bajaj, the researchers describe "EncephalApp", a smartphone-based application that allows patients and caregivers to conduct weekly point-of-care cognitive testing to assess for worsening HE, which traditionally was only performed by health care professionals.[44] Although the investigators acknowledge that longitudinal data on HE readmission rates are not yet available, they nevertheless highlight the potential benefits of having a valid assessment tool to screen for HE that can be quickly and easily administered at home without the need for a health care provider.[44,45] Ultimately, empowering patients with the tools to track progression in their disease enables them to promptly alert their health care team, which allows health care providers to intervene before disease severity escalates to the extent that hospitalization is necessary.

DISCUSSION

Since the recognition nearly 20 years ago of hospital readmissions as a major problem for patients with HE, multiple interventions have been developed and proven to reduce these readmissions. The next step is scaling them to clinical practice nationwide. One limitation to scalability is misaligned financial incentives—reducing readmissions primarily financially benefits payers, not the providers and hospitals that would implement them. Fortunately, this limitation is starting to be offset by the rise of value-based care reimbursement mechanisms. Several other financial incentives exist, such as the Medicare all-cause readmission incentive, as well as local partnerships with commercial payers.

In summary, hospital readmissions in patients with cirrhosis are common, costly, and associated with worse outcomes. Multiple proven strategies exist to reduce readmissions, which can be deployed in the inpatient, immediate postdischarge, or longitudinal community setting.

DISCLOSURE

None.

REFERENCES

1. Tapper EB, Halbert B, Mellinger J. Rates of and reasons for hospital readmissions in patients with cirrhosis: a multistate population-based cohort study. Clin Gastroenterol Hepatol 2016;14(8):1181–1188 e2.
2. Sood KT, Wong RJ. Hepatic encephalopathy is a strong predictor of early hospital readmission among cirrhosis patients. J Clin Exp Hepatol 2019;9(4):484–90.
3. Scaglione SJ, Metcalfe L, Kliethermes S, et al. Early hospital readmissions and mortality in patients with decompensated cirrhosis enrolled in a large national health insurance administrative database. J Clin Gastroenterol 2017;51(9): 839–44.
4. Desai AP, Satoskar R, Appannagari A, et al. Co-management between hospitalist and hepatologist improves the quality of care of inpatients with chronic liver disease. J Clin Gastroenterol 2014;48(4):e30–6.
5. Tapper EB, Hao S, Lin M, et al. The quality and outcomes of care provided to patients with cirrhosis by advanced practice providers. Hepatology 2020;71(1): 225–34.
6. Shaw J, Beyers L, Bajaj JS. Inadequate practices for hepatic encephalopathy management in the inpatient setting. J Hosp Med 2022;17(Suppl 1):S8–16.
7. Thomson MJ, Lok ASF, Tapper EB. Appropriate and potentially inappropriate medication use in decompensated cirrhosis. Hepatology 2021;73(6):2429–40.
8. Hayward KL, Patel PJ, Valery PC, et al. Medication-related problems in outpatients with decompensated cirrhosis: opportunities for harm prevention. Hepatol Commun 2019;3(5):620–31.
9. March KL, Peters MJ, Finch CK, et al. Pharmacist transition-of-care services improve patient satisfaction and decrease hospital readmissions. J Pharm Pract 2022;35(1):86–93.
10. Shull MT, Braitman LE, Stites SD, et al. Effects of a pharmacist-driven intervention program on hospital readmissions. Am J Health Syst Pharm 2018;75(9):e221–30.
11. Nardelli S, Lattanzi B, Merli M, et al. Muscle alterations are associated with minimal and overt hepatic encephalopathy in patients with liver cirrhosis. Hepatology 2019;70(5):1704–13.
12. Montano-Loza AJ, Angulo P, Meza-Junco J, et al. Sarcopenic obesity and myosteatosis are associated with higher mortality in patients with cirrhosis. J Cachexia Sarcopenia Muscle 2016;7(2):126–35.
13. Tapper EB, Finkelstein D, Mittleman MA, et al. A quality improvement initiative reduces 30-day rate of readmission for patients with cirrhosis. Clin Gastroenterol Hepatol 2016;14(5):753–9.
14. Louissaint J, Grzyb K, Bashaw L, et al. An electronic decision support intervention reduces readmissions for patients with cirrhosis. Am J Gastroenterol 2022; 117(3):491–4.
15. Kripalani S, Chen G, Ciampa P, et al. A transition care coordinator model reduces hospital readmissions and costs. Contemp Clin Trials 2019;81:55–61.

16. Garrido M, Turco M, Formentin C, et al. An educational tool for the prophylaxis of hepatic encephalopathy. BMJ Open Gastroenterol 2017;4(1):e000161.

17. Volk ML. Hospital readmissions for decompensated cirrhosis. Clin Liver Dis 2014; 4(6):138–40.

18. Yoder L, Mladenovic A, Pike F, et al. Attendance at a transitional liver clinic may Be associated with reduced readmissions for patients with liver disease. Am J Med 2022;135(2):235–43.e2.

19. Kimer N, Krag A, Møller S, et al. Systematic review with meta-analysis: the effects of rifaximin in hepatic encephalopathy. Aliment Pharmacol Ther 2014;40(2): 123–32.

20. Bass NM, Mullen KD, Sanyal A, et al. Rifaximin treatment in hepatic encephalopathy. N Engl J Med 2010;362(12):1071–81.

21. Mullen KD, Sanyal AJ, Bass NM, et al. Rifaximin is safe and well tolerated for long-term maintenance of remission from overt hepatic encephalopathy. Clin Gastroenterol Hepatol 2014;12(8):1390–7.e2.

22. Neff G, Zachry W III. Systematic review of the economic burden of overt hepatic encephalopathy and pharmacoeconomic impact of rifaximin. Pharmacoeconomics 2018;36(7):809–22.

23. Bajaj JS, Sanyal AJ, Bell D, et al. Predictors of the recurrence of hepatic encephalopathy in lactulose-treated patients. Aliment Pharmacol Ther 2010;31(9): 1012–7.

24. Rosenblatt R, Yeh J, Gaglio PJ. Long-Term management: modern measures to prevent readmission in patients with hepatic encephalopathy. Clin Liver Dis 2020;24(2):277–90.

25. Leise MD, Poterucha JJ, Kamath PS, et al. Management of hepatic encephalopathy in the hospital. Mayo Clin Proc 2014;89(2):241–53.

26. Kini V, Ho PM. Interventions to improve medication adherence: a review. JAMA 2018;320(23):2461–73.

27. Conn VS, Ruppar TM, Chan KC, et al. Packaging interventions to increase medication adherence: systematic review and meta-analysis. Curr Med Res Opin 2015;31(1):145–60.

28. Bajaj JS, Lauridsen M, Tapper EB, et al. Important unresolved questions in the management of hepatic encephalopathy: an ISHEN consensus. Am J Gastroenterol 2020;115(7):989–1002.

29. Frenette CT, Levy C, Saab S. Hepatic encephalopathy-related hospitalizations in cirrhosis: transition of care and closing the revolving door. Dig Dis Sci 2022;67(6): 1994–2004.

30. Riegler G, Esposito I. Bristol scale stool form. A still valid help in medical practice and clinical research. Tech Coloproctol 2001;5(3):163–4.

31. Lewis SJ, Heaton KW. Stool form scale as a useful guide to intestinal transit time. Scand J Gastroenterol 1997;32(9):920–4.

32. Vandeputte D, Falony G, Vieira-Silva S, et al. Stool consistency is strongly associated with gut microbiota richness and composition, enterotypes and bacterial growth rates. Gut 2016;65(1):57–62.

33. Duong NH, Bajaj D. Lactulose may not pass the "Acid" test in Hepatic Encephalopathy. Clin Gastroenterol Hepatol 2021.

34. Sharma S, Chauhan A. Use of lactulose in hepatic encephalopathy: is it time to shift targets? Clin Gastroenterol Hepatol 2022;20(5):e1220–1.

35. Bajaj JS, Ridlon JM, Hylemon PB, et al. Linkage of gut microbiome with cognition in hepatic encephalopathy. Am J Physiol Gastrointest Liver Physiol 2012;302(1): G168–75.

36. Ahluwalia V, Wade JB, Moeller FG, et al. The etiology of cirrhosis is a strong deter-minant of brain reserve: a multimodal magnetic resonance imaging study. Liver Transpl 2015;21(9):1123–32.

37. Bajaj JS, Kassam Z, Fagan A, et al. Fecal microbiota transplant from a rational stool donor improves hepatic encephalopathy: a randomized clinical trial. Hepa-tology 2017;66(6):1727–38.

38. Morando F, Maresio G, Piano S, et al. How to improve care in outpatients with cirrhosis and ascites: a new model of care coordination by consultant hepatolo-gists. J Hepatol 2013;59(2):257–64.

39. Tapper EB, Volk M. Strategies to reduce 30-day readmissions in patients with cirrhosis. Curr Gastroenterol Rep 2017;19(1):1.

40. Morales BP, Planas R, Bartoli R, et al. HEPACONTROL. A program that reduces early readmissions, mortality at 60 days, and healthcare costs in decompensated cirrhosis. Dig Liver Dis 2018;50(1):76–83.

41. Vadhariya A, Chen H, Serna O, et al. A retrospective study of drug utilization and hospital readmissions among Medicare patients with hepatic encephalopathy. Medicine (Baltim) 2020;99(16):e19603.

42. Thakkar J, Kurup R, Laba TL, et al. Mobile telephone text messaging for medica-tion adherence in chronic disease: a meta-analysis. JAMA Intern Med 2016; 176(3):340–9.

43. Ganapathy D, Acharya C, Lachar J, et al. The patient buddy app can potentially prevent hepatic encephalopathy-related readmissions. Liver Int 2017;37(12): 1843–51.

44. Bajaj JS, Thacker LR, Heuman DM, et al. The Stroop smartphone application is a short and valid method to screen for minimal hepatic encephalopathy. Hepatol-ogy 2013;58(3):1122–32.

45. Tapper EB, Parikh ND, Waljee AK, et al. Diagnosis of minimal hepatic encepha-lopathy: a systematic review of point-of-care diagnostic tests. Am J Gastroenterol 2018;113(4):529–38.

Moving?

Make sure your subscription moves with you!

To notify us of your new address, find your **Clinics Account Number** (located on your mailing label above your name), and contact customer service at:

Email: journalscustomerservice-usa@elsevier.com

800-654-2452 (subscribers in the U.S. & Canada)
314-447-8871 (subscribers outside of the U.S. & Canada)

Fax number: 314-447-8029

**Elsevier Health Sciences Division
Subscription Customer Service
3251 Riverport Lane
Maryland Heights, MO 63043**

*To ensure uninterrupted delivery of your subscription, please notify us at least 4 weeks in advance of move.

ELSEVIER

Printed and bound by CPI Group (UK) Ltd, Croydon, CR0 4YY

03/10/2024

01040470-0014